DO YOU KNOW THE ANSWERS TO THESE QUESTIONS?

- Why does a 22-year-o̶ al hair that she spends 20 m before she is willing to leave
- Why does a 24-year-ol̶ ̶ ̶ ̶ ̶ periods two or more months apart? Will it affect her ability to conceive?
- Why does a 37-year-old college teacher gain 60 pounds in one year and stop getting her periods?
- Why does a 32-year-old sales representative still get painful acne that sometimes leaves scars?
- Why does an attractive 48-year-old homemaker suddenly lose so much hair that she refuses to go to social gatherings?
- Why does a 28-year-old bride find herself experiencing mood swings since she started taking birth control pills?
- Why does a 3-year-old start to develop breasts—to her parents' great alarm?
- Why does a 54-year-old attorney who just started estrogen replacement now feel nauseated in the morning in a way that reminds her of being pregnant?

THESE WOMEN AND GIRLS HAVE PROBLEMS RELATED TO FEMALE HORMONES. THEY NEED ESSENTIAL INFORMATION AND SAFE, EFFECTIVE TREATMENT. NOW, *YOU* CAN GET THE FACTS IN—

THE GOOD NEWS ABOUT WOMEN'S HORMONES

GEOFFREY REDMOND, M.D., president of the Foundation for Developmental Endocrinology, Inc., graduated from Cornell, received an M.A. from the University of Virginia, an M.D. from Columbia, and did post-doctoral work at Columbia and Rockefeller universities. He has treated thousands of women and children with hormonal disorders at The Women's Hormone Center, his Beachwood, Ohio, clinic. Editor of two medical textbooks, he is also the author of eighty medical articles. Dr. Redmond has lectured throughout the United States and in eleven foreign countries.

THE GOOD NEWS ABOUT

WOMEN'S HORMONES

COMPLETE INFORMATION AND PROVEN SOLUTIONS FOR THE MOST COMMON HORMONAL PROBLEMS

GEOFFREY REDMOND, M.D.

WARNER BOOKS

A Time Warner Company

Copyright © 1995 by Geoffrey P. Redmond, M.D.
All rights reserved.

Warner Books, Inc., 1271 Avenue of the Americas, New York, NY 10020

Ⓦ A Time Warner Company

Printed in the United States of America
First Printing: May 1995
10 9 8 7 6 5 4 3

Library of Congress Cataloging-in-Publication Data

Redmond, Geoffrey P.
   The good news about women's hormones : complete information and proven solutions for the most common hormonal problems / Geoffrey Redmond.
       p.   cm.
   Includes bibliographical references and index.
   ISBN 0-446-39454-8
   1. Endocrine gynecology—Popular works.   2. Endocrine glands—Diseases—Popular works.   I. Title.
   RG159.R43   1995
   618.1—dc20   94-18095
                                                                  CIP

Cover design by Susan Newman
Book design by Giorgetta Bell McRee

To my teachers,
and most of all to my patients,
whose willingness to talk openly
about their hormonal problems
has taught me most of all.

Contents

Contents

List of Illustrations

Acknowledgments

In the course of the long path to becoming a doctor one depends so much on the generosity of one's teachers that it is daunting to try to remember and acknowledge all to whom one has a debt. I am sure I have left out many who should be here and hope that any who should read this work will not take their omission as lack of gratitude.

I must begin with Aaron Bannett, M.D., without whose interest in me and nurturing of my tentative beginnings of interest in medicine I would never have become a physician. Throughout my life he has been an example for me of the ideally dedicated physician.

Several of my teachers took my youthful interest in science seriously and encouraged me, especially Anthony Keasby and William Williams at Riverdale School.

George Perera, M.D., accepted me for medical school at P & S and provided benign supervision for my years there. Professor Gerald Cohen gave me my start in research, and my first work on male/female differences was done under his guidance and encouragement. I have never known anyone more enthusiastic about scientific research nor more willing to encourage those just beginning it.

I was privileged to work in the laboratory of Doctors Bruce McEwen and Lewis Krey at Rockefeller University, where I was trained in the basic science of reproductive endocrinology.

The late Albert Grokoest, M.D., set an example for me as he did for so many others of the physician who is at home in the humanities as in the sciences and always concerned about his patients as people.

I owe more to my teachers in pediatric endocrinology— Doctors Akira Morishima, M.D., and Jennifer Bell, M.D.— than I have ever expressed to them. Soja Bennett, M.D., taught me to read bone age X rays, a skill which I have used ever since. My knowledge of adult endocrinology was greatly enlarged by members of that division at the University of Vermont, especially Doctors Ethan A. Sims, Edward Horton, and Elliot Danforth. From them I learned much about insulin resistance and diabetes as well as benefiting from the example of their critical approach to medical science. Mrs. Dorothea Sims taught me the importance a positive approach has for those living with a medical condition. Lester F. Soyka, then and since, has fostered my interest in clinical pharmacology, the study of how medications affect human patients, and his advice has been of immeasurable value to me as has his friendship.

O. Peter Schumacher, M.D., recruited me for the Cleveland Clinic where I served from 1982 to 1990. He encouraged my interest in androgenic disorders and female endocrinology and shared unselfishly with me his enormous fund of clinical knowledge. I also learned much from and enjoyed collegial relationships with Doctors Angelo Licata, Leslie Sheeler, and Larry Kohse.

I must particularly mention Doctor Wilma Bergfeld. I remember well our first meeting in the Doctors' cafeteria at the Cleveland Clinic and discussing with her the possibility of collaborating on work in androgenic disorders. This small beginning led to our developing what is probably the largest

Introduction

*T*here has been an enormous need for a book about female hormonal disorders that would make this group of conditions understandable to the several million American women who have them. Such a book needs to explain these conditions very clearly, because the medical literature on the subject confuses even endocrinologists, a group of physicians reputed to understand subtleties of physiology beyond the grasp of most other specialists. It would have to be written clearly and avoid the condescending attitude that in the past has often characterized the medical profession's approach to these specially female conditions. Many doctors are sympathetic and tactful. Some are not.

For instance, women who do not menstruate every month are told, "Nothing is wrong with you." Although well intended, such remarks do not reassure a woman who knows perfectly well that having periods several months apart is not normal. Or a woman may be told her problem is "just your hormones," as if a statement that vague explained anything.

1

Often patients are told that treatment is unnecessary or that the problem is not serious enough to be addressed. Or treatment may be given; for example, an oral contraceptive to regulate irregular periods, without any explanation of the cause or rationale of the treatment.

Some women see several doctors without getting anything better than this. Eventually they become demoralized about the possibility of ever understanding what is wrong and receiving help. Others read well-intentioned but inaccurate articles in lay publications and become frightened or demoralized. All this is especially sad because it is totally unnecessary. Hormonal problems can be understood, and almost all can be helped with safe medication or other treatments. There *is* good news about women's hormones.

My experience with the more than 3,000 women with androgenic disorders whom I have seen personally in my practice is, so far as I know, the largest in the world. I also see many women with the full range of female hormone problems: too few or too many periods, menopause, abnormal pubertal development, obesity, fatigue, fluid retention, mood changes, and weight problems. I also see young girls with problems related to their development.

I have conducted my practice so that the data acquired during the very complete evaluation we do for each patient is combined so as to be able to improve knowledge about these conditions. My past laboratory research experience has enabled me to select laboratories that can do difficult hormone assays precisely. I have treated the same patients and followed them for up to eleven years. Much of the data has been put into a computer database and analyzed with the aid of expert biostatisticians.

All this has meant that I—and those who have worked with me—have had the best possible opportunity to learn about female endocrinology not simply from books and journals, important as these are, but from the real women who are doing their best to actually live with hormonal disorders. This unique experience has made it possible to correlate what happens to hormones in the blood with what happens in the patient's body and in her life. For me, this has been an exciting opportunity to combine the technical and human sides of medicine. I have learned from radioimmunoassays, from computer-generated graphs, from sophisticated imaging techniques. And I have also learned from listening to my patients, hearing their stories, and inviting them to share their feelings about the changes in their bodies that brought them to me.

I think I have also learned how to explain hormonal conditions in ways that are not only medically sound but also respectful of the affected person's dignity. Some of the women who came to me were initially shy or defensive because they had experienced derogatory treatment by other physicians. Women with increased facial hair are often told they have "too many male hormones." Some who have thinning scalp hair are told it is "just because you are getting old." Some of my patients with irregular periods have been told, in effect, "Don't worry about it, but you probably won't be able to get pregnant." Usually this advice is invalid as well as being unfeeling.

Other doctors try to explain but do not define the technical terms they use. Endocrinology has more than its share of such terms; even for other health professionals, translation is essential. Talking in biochemical terms can make an explanation seem remote from a problem. My approach in this book is to talk not about hormones by themselves, but as they affect women's lives.

In this book, I cannot answer your questions directly, but I have tried my best to think of any questions you might ask and to give the answers. Because I spend so much of my time talking to women about their hormones, I have a good idea of what your questions are likely to be. Still, I may have left out something that is important for you to know. A book cannot substitute for your own doctor. But it should help make the interaction with your doctor more valuable for you by giving you vital information that there may not be time to discuss or that might be forgotten while you are in his or her office.

How to Help This Book Help You

If you have a hormone problem or if someone important to you does, this book is for you. You may have irregular periods, your mother may be menopausal, or your daughter may seem to be developing too early. You may have more intense mood swings than are comfortable for you during the week before your period is due. Or your concern may be one or more of the many other conditions discussed in this book.

The purpose of the book is to give you all the information you need to understand the condition, why it is happening to you, what possible harm it might cause, and what the treatment options are. You might also just be curious because you know hormones are important to a woman's well-being and want to understand them better.

If you are willing to take the time to read a book like this, you deserve certain commitments from me. I will do my best to be clear and avoid mystification. Certain of the effects of hormones, such as the transformation of a girl's body into that of a woman, will always have some mystery about them. But the biological aspects need not be mysterious. I also promise to discuss the effects of these conditions in a manner that is straightforward but not demeaning. When your body is being discussed, tact and sensitivity are what you are entitled to. I will discuss all the available treatments for each condition, explain why they work and how well they work, and tell you about their side effects or risks. The discussions of risk include not only those of being treated but those of not being treated.

I will not withhold information about toxicity to induce you to take medication, but neither will I withhold information about the risks you take if you decide against treatment. This book will not make you able to be your own doctor, but it will tell you everything necessary for you to be sure you are being treated properly.

I ask certain things of you in return. One is that you be open-minded. Many of the new discoveries about hormones contradict old ideas. The word "hormone" has become fearful to some women and tends to raise the specter of cancer or other terrible ill effects. If you decide not to take hormones when I think they might be good for you, that is your right. But at least consider the information I have assembled here for you before making up your mind. I also ask that you consider this a book to be read, not merely a reference book for looking something up.

I have chosen to relate the stories of actual women with hormone problems (with appropriate alterations to protect privacy) because medical conditions are not entries in textbooks but problems that affect people's lives. I cover all the *common* female hormone problems, but not all the *possible* ones, because I think a complete discussion of the ones that are most likely to affect a woman's life is more useful than a series of brief entries, as in a medical dictionary.

I have given much more attention to how hormones affect the lives of women than to biochemistry, though that is here as well. That I have emphasized the human dimension does not mean that I have watered down the science. As an active researcher in the field, I have made the best effort I can to include all relevant scientific information, and to make it completely up to date, even including information not yet published and known only to "insiders" in the field of female endocrinology. This kind of information is especially important in rapidly advancing areas such as hormone replacement in menopause, because promising new approaches may not appear in medical journals until a year or more after they become known to researchers in the field.

Some of the information in this book has been known until now only to a handful of specialists. Much of it has never appeared in a lay publication. I have, of course, also included basic information that is not new but is necessary for you to have a balanced understanding of a topic.

The Good News About Women's Hormones was written in the belief that advances in endocrinology have the potential for eliminating the difficulties that so many women have had with hormonal problems in the past. In the 1990s, women no longer need be prisoners of their hormones.

Finding the Right Doctor for Female Hormone Problems

Although it has considerable problems, the American health-care system is far and away the best in the world. Apart from cost, the greatest problem people face in getting the care they need is locating the right doctor. Whatever your medical problem, there is almost certainly someone who is very knowledgeable and experienced in that area. The following is some general advice to help you find out who it is.

Our system has two extremes. The famous institutions tend to be geared to the needs of researchers or to critically ill patients rather than to those whose problems, like most female hormonal disorders, are disturbing, unpleasant, sometimes embarrassing, but rarely life-threatening. Physicians in primary care and HMOs tend to the other extreme: They provide care mainly for common conditions but ignore more subtle ones if they are not life-threatening. To find the best care for your hormonal problem you may have to be assertive. If you are in an HMO or other managed-care plan, insist that the problem is serious to you and that you expect referral to a specialist. If you can chose your physician, do some research into who in your community is competent in these areas.

Several categories of specialists treat female hormone problems. Reproductive endocrinologists are gynecologists who have done advanced study in female hormone problems and infertility. Standards in this subspecialty are high, and most who achieve board certification are highly skilled. Most, however, emphasize infertility rather than the non-pregnancy aspects of the conditions described in this book. The professional organization for reproductive endocrinologists is the American Fertility Society, which also includes physicians of other specialties, as well as laboratory scientists.

Medical endocrinologists have first specialized in internal medicine or occasionally, like myself, in pediatrics before doing two to three years of further training in hormonal disorders. However, interests of endocrinologists vary, and not all are experienced in female hormone problems. The primary professional organization for this subspecialty is the Endocrine Society, which includes researchers as well as clinicians.

For children, it is best to find a board-certified pediatric endocrinologist. Some adult endocrinologists will treat children, but they rarely understand the subtleties of growth and development or pubertal disorders. The professional organization for pediatric endocrinology is the Lawson Wilkins Pediatric Endocrine Society.

Most people with acne first consult a dermatologist. Standards in this specialty are high. However, most dermatologists are not experienced with hormonal treatment of acne or hair-growth problems. If you think hormonal treatment is a consideration for your condition, it is reasonable to first make a phone call to ask if a particular dermatologist is willing to provide this form of therapy.

It is best to get recommendations from doctors or other

health professionals in your community, then call the office of the doctor in question and ask if he or she treats many patients with the condition you are concerned about. If the answer is no, then more inquiry may be warranted. An alternative is to call the department of endocrinology or gynecology at a nearby medical school and ask who in the department has a special interest in the condition you have. Minimal qualifications are board certification in reproductive endocrinology, endocrinology, or pediatric endocrinology, and membership in the relevant specialty society. In the resource guide at the end of this book, I have listed the main professional organizations concerned with female hormone problems, as well as lay groups. Some of the latter can give advice and support for women with hormonal disorders.

The chances are that you will need a specialist to get the kind of understanding you will need. Surprisingly little is taught to medical students about women's special hormonal makeup, even in the advanced training programs of many specialties. Yet virtually all doctors have women patients and need at least a general knowledge of how hormones affect them. The result is that women often have difficulty finding a doctor who understands their hormonal problems.

One reason for the tendency of medicine to ignore these conditions has to do with the habits of doctors and medical scientists. Doctors and scientists like objectivity, and hormone problems tend to seem subjective. It is easy to study a treatment for high blood pressure or high cholesterol levels because these things are easy to measure. But how does one measure a decrease in facial hair or an improvement in mood? What is most important is hardest to measure: the improvement in self-esteem or quality of life that results, say, from facial hair becoming less noticeable.

Using the Information in This Book About Medications

In this book, I discuss the important hormonal medications in great detail. My women patients want to know exactly what they are taking, why I have recommended it over the alternatives, what effects it will have on their bodies, and what possible adverse effects can occur. They also want to know how well and how quickly it will work. All these questions are reasonable and proper. I have tried to provide the answers to all these questions for each medication. Because the dose of a medication is as important as what the medication is, I have been explicit as to which doses are needed to be effective and which are excessive. Many medications have completely different effects at different doses, and this is especially true for hormones.

Often I have given ranges of doses rather than a single one because doses of hormones nearly always have to be individualized. A variety of factors affect dose, including weight, age (especially for children and for adults over sixty), other drugs being taken, and individual differences in metabolism. For this reason, I've given information about how doses are selected and adjusted.

My purpose in being so specific is definitely not to encourage you to treat yourself. This is unwise even if you are a physician. However, I do think you should be an active participant in your treatment. This means verifying and extending your understanding of the instructions the doctor gave you when she or he prescribed the hormones or other medications. You may well think of additional questions after you have left the doctor's office, and the answers to these will probably be in this book. While I do not think you should self-treat, I do think you should verify that the treatments prescribed for you are correct; more than that, that they are the best ones available in the current state of medical knowledge. It is no secret that doctors vary in how current they are in a particular area or how experienced they are with a specific condition. At least half of the women I see for the kinds of problems described in this book have seen one, or in some cases, several other physicians without being able to find an effective treatment. This is not as it should be, because our present state of knowledge about female hormone problems is quite good, and if you have one of the conditions I discuss in this book, the odds are that an effective treatment exists for it.

If you are not getting better and you are not being treated as described in this book, you may want to discuss the situation with your doctor or even seek a second opinion. Of course, there may be factors that make your condition different from any I have described here. If so, your doctor should be willing to explain this to you to your satisfaction. Your body is too important to you. You owe it to yourself as well as to those who care about you to get the best medical care available.

Many factors influence the choice of medications and their dose, so there may be some factor present in your case that I neglect to mention. Sometimes new information makes a particular point obsolete. Medicine is too complex and evolves too fast for there to be any final authority, including this book. This is why you need to discuss any concerns with a physician who knows your individual situation.

This book is meant to be practical so that you can participate in finding solutions to any hormonal problems you may have. To this end, I have given specific names of different preparations of hormones and other medications. This represents my own experience and opinion, though in most cases such information reflects a consensus among physicians about them. When there is controversy, I have explained the differing viewpoints and pointed out what I feel is most likely to be the correct one and why. I have also recommended specific preparations when several are available. I feel it is not fair to you to do otherwise. If I feel one medication is better, there is no reason to withhold this very useful information from you. At the same time, however, my purpose is to guide you in making choices, not to endorse specific products. In some cases, I recommend a product because I am familiar with it and know it is good; yet there may be others just as good that I do not know about, or something new may have come out after this book was published. I have given good choices, but not always the only choice. This is especially true when I discuss cosmetics and other over-the-counter products. However, if I do not recommend specific products, it may be difficult for you to find what you need among the large number of choices available.

In discussing drugs, I have followed standard medical writing practice in referring to them by generic rather than brand names, even though the latter are often more familiar. In each case, I have given the brand name at the beginning of the discussion of each medication. The exception is birth control pills, which I do refer to by brand name; using generic names of the two hormones in each pill would be too confusing.

In this book, I discuss many kinds of medication for the entire range of female hormone problems. I want it to be very clear to all my readers, however, that I do not see medication as the answer to every problem. In many cases, illnesses correct themselves if we simply wait. In other cases, changes in nutrition and lifestyle are the best solution. These matters are discussed throughout this book and especially in Chapter Nine. However, there are many situations in which medication is the best answer, and these are the kinds of problems about which people are likely to consult a physician. So a medical book inevitably spends much of its time on pharmacologic approaches to ills. These are also the treatments about which it is hardest for lay people to get solid information. The extensive discussion of drugs, their uses, and side effects reflects the need to give you adequate information about them, not a preference on my part for drugs over non-drug alternatives when they exist.

The best way to test a drug is by controlled studies on large numbers of people. Many of the treatments discussed in this book have been tested in this way, but some have not. For example, there are few studies comparing the effects of different hormone preparations to each other. Most simply compare different doses of the same preparation. The most conservative doctors will not even consider the possibility that a drug has a benefit until it has been rigorously proved in large-scale clinical trials. However, there are two big problems with this skeptical attitude. One is that it takes years for these kinds of studies to be done. Most conditions cannot wait this long. Another is cost: The cheapest clinical trials cost a few hundred thousand dollars, and the most expensive cost several million. For many applications of drugs, there is just no one who is willing to pay for it. However, all medications have had very extensive testing extending over several years before their release is approved by the Food and Drug Administration. While there is always more to be learned and always areas of uncertainty (which I will point out as I consider the different hormones), medicine has achieved an excellent knowledge base concerning hormones.

Many of the women who come to see me are interested in whether there are any non-drug treatments for their conditions. When there are effective non-drug alternatives, I have described them in this book. However, a problem with non-conventional treatments such as vitamins and herbs is that there is usually a lack of objective evidence as to their efficacy. Anyone who has inquired into the subject becomes convinced that there is value to at least some alternative medical approaches, but as a physician I am reluctant to recommend a treatment until I see strong evidence that it is safe and effective.

For many alternative therapies, there is no data at all on whether they work and whether they are safe, other than the claims of their advocates. For this reason, one should be cautious about using non-conventional treatments.

Some nutritional therapies are clearly not sufficient by themselves. For example, calcium without estrogen does not prevent osteoporosis. Calcium supplementation is important for women, but it is not enough by itself. I am sure that the next decade will bring better information about non-conventional therapies and that as a result they will come to have a larger place in medical practice.

When research started to produce new and effective drugs in the 1940s and 1950s, people were eager to take each new "wonder drug." Unfortunate experiences with unanticipated side effects have made us all more cautious. Some mistakes were made with hormonal treatments in those early days, and some still fear them for that reason. Before deciding to take any medication, you should inform yourself about it and consider carefully. However, automatically avoiding medication is not the best way to protect yourself. The safety of a drug resides not only in the medication itself, but also in how well and carefully it is used. A drug that sounds dangerous may be safe if properly monitored. Individual differences are important also. A drug must be understood in the context of its use and of the person taking it. I have discussed these individual factors in considerable detail to aid you in making the best choices for yourself.

You must also consider the reason for taking a drug. When there is no need to take a drug, it is not worth any risk to take it. When it has the possibility of improving an important aspect of your life, it may be worth putting up with side effects. There are often ways their impact can be minimized, and they are not necessarily unalterable.

Like clothes, medications must fit the person taking them.

Drugs are not just for diseases, they are for people. Much of the progress in contemporary endocrinology is in understanding the differences in the responses to medications.

I have discussed these issues concerning medications as a background for more specific discussion of the different hormones. We need to consider hormones in two aspects: as substances naturally present in the body and affecting its functioning, and/or as substances taken as medication to correct these processes when they are not functioning normally. The next chapter explains the hormones themselves. Later chapters consider their roles in the various hormonal conditions that can affect women.

Chapter One

•

Some Women and Their Hormone Problems

*S*haron is a twenty-eight-year-old, single secretary. While in college, she became concerned about the amount of facial hair that had started growing on her upper lip and chin. Although a boy she once dated in college made a remark about her having a moustache, she thinks most people do not notice. To be certain that they will not, Sharon spends up to fifteen minutes each morning removing hairs before she can put on her makeup and leave for work. Each afternoon she must spend additional time replacing her makeup to be sure no one can see the hair growing back. She dresses attractively and has no shortage of dates, but resents the extra time she must spend each morning and afternoon removing facial hair. She asked her gynecologist about it once, and he told her that her facial hair is "normal." Sharon does not agree that it is normal and was very interested when I explained to her that hair growth in women is controlled by hormones and that with blood tests we would be able to find out which ones were causing her problem. She was even more interested when I told her that this information would make it possible to select a treatment that was almost certain to be effective in decreasing her facial and body hair.

Lenore is thirty-one years old and a computer programmer. She has also noticed more hair on her upper lip than was there when she graduated from college. But what really bothers her is that her face is always broken out. It began as teenage acne when she was fifteen, but just about the time her friends' complexions were clearing up in their late teens, hers was getting worse. Lenore's mother took her to a dermatologist when she was in high school. Several topical medications were prescribed, but she often forgot to use them. She now gets large, red, painful areas on her face that she refers to as boils. Often these leave small scars that do not go away. Over the last few years, her once-smooth skin has become pitted.

Lenore saw another dermatologist at a university medical center. He prescribed an oral antibiotic and several creams that she applied to her face morning and evening. This time, she followed the doctor's instructions exactly. With the medication, Lenore did not have quite as many pimples, but the boils continued to appear, and she still felt embarrassed by the pitting in her skin. She was still afraid to be in situations, like swimming, in which she was likely to be seen without her makeup. Lenore thought, correctly, that her acne must be coming from some internal disorder, even though it was only her skin that was affected. She'd been told at various times that it was too much greasy food (by her friends) or that it was stress (by her family doctor). But she didn't notice any improvement when she cut down on her fat intake and didn't think she was really under more stress than other women she knew without acne. She agreed with enthusiasm when I told her it was time for her acne to clear up and that treatment directed at the cause—her hormones—would clear her skin far more effectively than antibiotics and creams.

*   *   *

Jennifer, a twenty-four-year-old student, came to see me at the suggestion of a friend who had been seeing me for a pituitary condition that had caused her to stop having periods. Jennifer's problem was milder; she had periods, but they came at least two months apart. This had been her pattern since her teens. She told me that although she worried that something might be wrong, she had always been too busy to pay much attention to it. She'd asked the gynecologist at the student health service why she did not have regular periods, but he simply told her it didn't matter unless she wanted to get pregnant. Jennifer recalled with some irritation that the gynecologist had been more concerned about whether she needed birth control than with her not getting her period. Jennifer had not thought of going to another doctor, but when she happened to tell her friend about her irregular cycle, her friend told her she'd had the same problem and had recommended that she see me. Testing showed that Jennifer had no serious hormonal disease; what she had was a common condition called hypothalamic amenorrhea. With this condition, the brain does not signal the pituitary gland to start the menstrual cycle each month. We discussed her excellent prospects for fertility, and Jennifer was finally able to understand why she was not getting her period.

Although three-year-old Tracey's problem was not an emergency, I had added her onto my schedule at short notice because her condition was one that is extremely disturbing to mothers. Tracey had started to develop breasts and pubic hair. Mothers often have mixed feelings when they see their daughters start to develop, since it marks the end of childhood. But when these normal events occur at the wrong age, a mother's reaction is shock and fear. Tracey's mother thought the breast development had begun four or five months earlier, but at first she had attributed it to weight gain. But when pubic hair started to appear, she knew that more was involved.

Tracey was actually starting to develop. Precocious puberty, the medical term for the appearance of breasts and pubic hair in a girl before age eight, is a well-recognized condition. I reassured her mother at once that the condition is treatable. I did not want her to worry any longer than necessary that she would be faced with handling menstrual periods in a three- or four-year-old girl. Yet that is exactly what can happen if this condition is left untreated.

Fortunately Tracey's workup did not reveal any of the serious causes of this disorder, such as a tumor of the brain or ovary. Treatment with a new kind of drug called a Gn-RH analogue was started, and over a few weeks the breast development became much less conspicuous. Tracey's mother was now able to stop worrying about how she could handle puberty in a three-year-old.

Patricia is thirty-seven and a hospital administrator. She came to me in near despair about not being able to control her weight. She weighed 270 pounds, 60 of which were gained in the last fourteen months. Her main concern was her weight, but she was also worried about her menstrual cycle. She told me that she had always missed two or three periods a year, but now they were even less frequent; in fact, the last one had been four months earlier. Because of her embarrassment about her weight, Patricia does not like to go to doctors and had almost decided she would just live with her strange periods. She also told me she had tried "all the diets there are," and none of them had worked.

Patricia had been told a few years earlier that her infrequent periods did not matter so long as she did not want to conceive. She suspected that the gynecologist assumed she was unlikely to get married because of her weight problem and that this was why he seemed uninterested in her menstrual abnormality.

Patricia was not even sure she wanted children. But she quite understandably resented being patronized and knew perfectly well she was missing periods because of a hormonal abnormality. She wanted to understand what this was and whether she needed any treatment for it. When I explained how weight gain affects female hormones, she was quite relieved to be able to understand the changes in her body, although of course she was still not happy about having gained weight. Nor did she really want to take medication to bring on her periods, but she was willing to do so when I explained that this would protect her against a form of female cancer (of the endometrium, the lining of the uterus) she was otherwise at risk for. As she told me, "I may not have gotten entirely good news today, but I needed to hear it."

We discussed a special diet that can facilitate weight loss in part by reversing one of the hormonal changes that makes it so hard for women to lose weight. This diet, called the PSMF (for protein-sparing modified fast), lowers the high insulin levels that are one factor preventing fat from being broken down. (I explain this diet in detail in Chapter Ten, "Being Overweight.") At that time she did not feel she could follow it, but she returned several months later, ready to give it a try.

Judy, age forty-eight, has raised three children. Prior to the birth of her first child, she worked in sales. Now she devotes considerable time to volunteer activities and to entertaining for social functions related to her husband's work as a corporate executive. Recently she has participated with increasing reluctance in these activities, which she once greatly enjoyed. About eight months before she came to see me, Judy noticed that her hair was thinner. She now finds a considerable amount of hair on the shoulders of her dresses and in the bathtub after showering. She became tearful as she related to me her fear that others will notice she is losing her hair. This now makes social functions she once would have enjoyed very stressful for her. Her husband has admitted to her that he can see a change, but he tells her that others will not notice or not care if they do. This does not reassure Judy at all. She told me that she was starting to worry about her marriage because her social schedule had become such a strain for her.

Although Judy has continued to get her periods regularly, I suspected that the hair loss might be a result of early estrogen deficiency because, for some women, hair loss is the first sign of menopause. Lack of estrogen is one of several hormone changes that can cause alopecia (the medical term for hair loss) in women. Because of her regular periods, Judy had not thought of this possibility. When I described a hot flash to her, she thought she had had some at night, but she had not paid them much attention. On reflection, she recalled that her periods had gotten a little lighter. Testing did indeed point to estrogen deficiency as the cause of Judy's hair loss, and treatment was able to restore nearly all of the lost hair, although it took several months of treatment for this to happen.

Not all women with hair loss are approaching menopause. Deanna, a twenty-eight-year-old, saw me for the same problem. She noticed that she was losing hair and that the back of her head was especially affected. She told me she felt uncomfortable in public situations because she feared people were staring at the back of her head. In Deanna's case, the cause of the hair loss was not lack of estrogen, but increased levels of a family of hormones called androgens. Treatment was also effective but required quite different medications than those that eased Judy's hair problem. Improvement took longer, but it did come.

Rebecca is a twenty-four-year-old whose mother had called me the week before her visit to discuss her daughter's problem. Her mother told me her daughter had been married seven months earlier. Though basically quite happy, Rebecca had noticed herself getting very moody and sought her mother's advice. Her mother had called to make the appointment for Rebecca but asked me not to tell her daughter she had talked to me because she did not want to seem to be meddling. The following week Rebecca came for her appointment. She was a pleasant and cheerful young woman, hardly someone I would have guessed, when I saw her sitting in my waiting room, to be troubled by mood swings. When she started to explain why she had come, her face showed real worry. She told me a little defensively that she was very happily married but very often found herself depressed and would start to cry for no reason. "Really, I love my husband," she said, "and everything at my job is fine. I just do not know why this is happening to me." As I went through her health history, I learned that she had begun the use of oral contraceptives two months before her marriage. The low moods began about a month after her wedding. The pill she took turned out to be one that is frequently prescribed but that contains a fairly high dose of the hormone norethindrone. This ingredient mimics the action of the natural hormone progesterone. High levels of this hormone cause a depressed mood, similar to what some women get just before their periods. Most women take this pill without any problems, but a few get depressed from it.

I explained this to Rebecca and suggested she change to another pill that has only 30 percent of the amount of this hormone as the pill she was on. Of course, I had asked her a little about her marriage because it is important to consider psychological factors in situations like this. But I was careful not to insist that her problem was in her head. Nothing does a greater disservice to a patient with a hormonal problem than to mistake it for a psychological one.

When I saw Rebecca for follow-up three months later, she greeted me with a big smile. She told me that the switch to the new pill had "changed everything." She no longer felt depressed and could enjoy her first year of marriage like any other newlywed. Correcting the problem involved only a simple medication change, but it did require a knowledge of how female hormones act on the brain.

Nor are problems with female hormone treatment confined to women using the pill. Another patient of mine had just started taking estrogen replacement, at the age of fifty-four, for menopause. The estrogen had been a major boost to her. She worked in a nearby city as a prosecuting attorney and before seeking treatment had found herself extremely embarrassed when she had a hot flash just as she was summing up a case to a jury. The hormonal medications, Premarin® (Wyeth-Ayerst) and Provera® (Upjohn), prescribed by her gynecologist, are standard ones and had taken away the hot flashes after two or three weeks. This had made a great difference to my patient, and she was quite grateful, even to the point of apologizing for having any complaints about the medications. But she had noticed that many mornings she felt nauseous. While she never actually vomited, the nausea made her quite uncomfortable. Yet she felt she needed the estrogen. Joking, she said that she almost wondered if she were pregnant again because the feeling reminded her so much of the morning sickness she had had with all three of her pregnancies. I explained that a rapid rise in estrogen makes many women nauseous until the brain gets used to the new level. We worked out a schedule for her to temporarily decrease the dose and gradually work back up to the level she had been taking. Although she did have some very mild hot flashes on the lower dose, these were less bothersome to her than the nausea, and they went away completely once she was back on the higher amount, this time without nausea.

What do all these women of differing ages and lifestyles have in common? At first glance, their problems—increased hair growth, adult acne, infrequent periods, early puberty, weight gain, hair loss, moodiness, and nausea—seem quite different. A few had been able to get partial help for their problems, but others had found the members of the medical profession generally unsympathetic to their concerns. Most have managed to do what they wanted in their lives despite the worry or embarrassment caused by their condition. But they all felt their quality of life was not what it should be. They were therefore quite willing to spend the time and money to go to a specialist in the hope of feeling better.

In this book, I will tell you what the science of endocrinology has learned about the diverse group of hormones that control the functioning of a woman's body. I will explain what they do in the body and how they sometimes cause unwanted changes: in mood, in appearance, in weight, in menstruation, in fertility. I will make clear how they cause disturbing alterations in hair growth. And I'll also tell you about new evidence that some abnormalities in female hormones can cause changes in cholesterol that may predispose women to heart attacks in later years.

But I would not expect you to take the time to learn about these things unless there was some practical benefit to you, the woman with a hormonal disorder. And so I will also tell you about newly developed laboratory techniques that permit accurate measurement of minute levels of hormones at acceptable cost, and how these tests can be used to pinpoint exactly what is happening with your hormones. Because such common problems as lack of menstruation, increased facial hair, or thinning of scalp hair can have different causes in different women, the tests are needed to individualize diagnosis and treatment. These tests can also make it possible to understand what is causing the problem. Living successfully with a condition starts with an understanding of what it is and how it affects your body. Often understanding makes almost as much difference as medication.

Lab tests alone do not make anyone better. So you may feel

that the most important parts of this book are the sections that describe how hormonal disorders can be successfully treated. Many women are afraid to take hormones. But the new knowledge described in this book can make it possible to design therapy so that risks are minimized or eliminated. And you can learn exactly what risks there are. You also will learn something sometimes left out of books and articles: what the risks are if you *do not* take medication. For example, the woman who does not menstruate normally may have later complications, depending on the levels of certain of her hormones. Proper medication can prevent this. The problems of persistent acne, increased hair growth, or scalp hair loss can be dramatically helped with medication. In general, these are safe and well tolerated, although they can have side effects. I will tell you not only what these medications are and how they can help, but what the side effects are and how you can deal with them. I will also tell you what you need to know to determine if you are someone who should avoid particular hormonal medications.

The existence of safe and effective treatments for female hormone problems makes it worth my time to write the book and your time to read it. All the women whose stories I have told were able to be helped, and I will return to them in the different chapters of this book. But far more than just a few women can be helped. In my experience, about 90 percent of women with female hormone problems can achieve substantial benefit with properly prescribed medications.

This book puts great emphasis on how hormones affect how a woman looks, because being satisfied with your appearance is part of a full and happy life. I am writing to give women with hormonal disorders the good news that there is help available. Hormonal disorders can be identified, their causes can be found, and effective treatment can be given. I am also writing for friends, spouses, relatives, and boyfriends of women with hormonal disorders, to help them understand the special problems these women face. And for doctors, too, in the hope that more will become interested in this group of conditions so that women will find help more easily available.

Too many women have been misled into believing that their hormones and the problems they sometimes cause are incomprehensible and intractable. Both ideas are wrong. There is no reason you cannot understand how your hormones affect your body. When hormones do things that are unwanted or unhealthy, something can almost always be done. As you will see from the stories of the women I tell you about, and from scientific information about treatments that are not only effective but safe, there is plenty of good news about women's hormones.

Hormonal disorders are common. The best estimates are that 10 percent of American women have irregular periods and that 5 percent have androgenic disorders, which can cause adult acne, increased facial and body hair, and scalp hair thinning. These estimates are conservative. For example, one survey showed that about 45 percent of American women remove unwanted facial hair at least occasionally. Obesity affects 40 percent of adults, and 10 to 20 percent of women are troubled by fluid retention. Hormonal disorders affect all races and demographic groups. There is no particular group or type of woman who gets a hormonal disorder. Such problems affect women of all races, married and single, young and old.

The true incidence of female hormonal problems tends to be underestimated, even by doctors, because affected women do their best to conceal their condition. By their nature, hormone problems tend to be intimate or embarrassing. Many women suffer quietly, having all but given up hope that anything can be done. This is both sad and unnecessary. Knowledge of endocrinology has advanced to the point where no woman should have to feel she is the prisoner of her hormones.

Chapter Two

•

Hormones: What They Are and How They Affect a Woman's Life

*Y*ou already know quite a lot about hormones because you experience their effects every day. Unlike other aspects of medicine that deal with processes mostly hidden from awareness, most of the effects of your hormones are ones you see or feel. Menstruation, for example, is the most hormonal of events in a woman's life. You already know the most important things about your cycle: when it began, how long it takes from one period to the next, how many days you bleed, how you feel at each stage, the relationship of the cycle to fertility. You even know something about the most commonly used hormonal medications, such as birth control pills. And you observe the effects of hormones in family members: the growth and maturation of your children and their friends, male and female development in teenagers, and sexuality in your romantic partner and yourself. This is what makes endocrinology interesting: While hormones are invisible, their effects are observable, and understanding them explains many of the most important ways our bodies function. Hormones are especially important in the processes in our bodies that change from day to day.

A key aspect of the good news that this book will emphasize is that you can understand your own hormones. In this chapter, I will do my best to explain the hormones themselves— their biochemical nature and how they act. In later chapters, I will explain how these hormones affect women's lives. Those chapters will focus more on the human aspects; this one is a little more abstract and scientific, but will give you factual information useful in understanding your body and your life. This is the purpose of medical science: to understand and improve the lives of actual people. Hormones are not merely chemicals in the blood; they are aspects of human experience.

Hormones cause problems when their levels are too high or too low. Sometimes the hormones themselves are normal, but the body's reaction to them is excessive. Then tests are less useful than physical examination for signs of the action of the relevant hormone. For example, all female acne is caused by the family of hormones called androgens. However, in many women with acne the androgen levels in the blood are normal, but the oil glands in their skin overreact to these normal levels. When you know how the various hormones act in your body, you will be able to figure out which ones may be causing your problem.

The word "hormone" comes from a Greek word meaning wanderer. Hormones are chemicals that journey through the bloodstream to all parts of the body. They are one of the two systems that coordinate the diverse cells and organs of the body; the other is the nervous system, whose connections to distant parts of the body are visible, at least to the anatomist. The nervous system seems to resemble a telephone system or a computer. The endocrine system is more like the weather; it operates by known principles but is never entirely predictable. Like weather, its effects are not precise, more a matter of mood than of cognition. For all their elusiveness, hormones are very powerful factors in our lives, especially through their involvement in the most dramatic aspects of our body's functioning: sexuality and reproduction.

In the decades after their discovery, hormones were almost regarded as miracle chemicals because of their ability to have such dramatic and diverse influence on the body. Later, when problems emerged in the medical use of hormones, their power seemed almost malign. Both concepts are outmoded. Medical scientists now think of hormones simply as substances that signal tissues to initiate events already programmed in them. Thus estrogen does not really have a mysterious power that causes the breasts to grow; rather it switches on processes of growth that are latent in the breast itself. The same is true for the dramatic effects of hormones on the mind at puberty. Testosterone does not in itself engender sexual feelings but activates the brain's capacity for desire.

Yet greater scientific knowledge about hormones has not robbed them of their fascination; their effects on our bodies and our lives are too great for them to be ignored. Whether this is more true of women than of men I do not know. I do know that women are more aware of their hormones which are more changeable in a woman's body and at times seem to wander around with a will of their own, producing effects a woman must live with. Many women have an ambivalent relationship to their hormones. Without them they would not be women, yet some of the processes the hormones control are disturbing or uncomfortable or embarrassing. Hormones are not only chemicals; they are daily events in women's lives.

What Are "Sex Steroid" Hormones?

Several of the hormones we will be considering are in the class known as "sex steroids." While this term is correct scientifically, it cannot avoid connotations of the erotic. This is one of the problems in understanding hormone problems; they become much more complicated—both to understand and to live with—because of their association with sexuality. But breasts, vaginas, and pubic hair are parts of the body like the heart, hands, and stomach. When health is the concern, they need to be considered with the same objectivity, even though we must also admit that they are in other ways not quite the same. A medical condition causing physical change related to sex and gender always has special emotional significance for the affected person. In scientific usage, however, a sex steroid is any one of a group of hormones belonging to the steroid chemical class and produced in the gonads (the general term for the glands of the reproductive system, the ovaries and testes). Sex steroids are also produced in the adrenal glands, which share some of their chemical activities with the gonads.

The term "steroid" by itself has also come into a common and misleading use that is somewhat different from scientific usage. In common speech, "steroids" has come to refer to the drugs sometimes used by athletes in the belief that they will increase their muscle bulk and thus their strength and performance. The full term for these is "anabolic steroid." It would have saved a lot of confusion if the slang term had been "anabolics" because that name refers to their distinctive effect of building up body tissue. While anabolics are indeed steroids, there are several other kinds of steroid hormones that are not like anabolics at all. The steroids are, in fact, a quite diverse family of substances that share a distinctive chemical core consisting of four interconnected rings of atoms. Steroids are all derived from cholesterol and have been adapted to regulation of bodily processes. Remember that to say a hormone or a drug is a steroid tells us about its chemical structure rather than its action in the body. When I use the term "steroid" in this book, it is a neutral one. Steroids are not good or bad, healthy or unhealthy as a group. Specific steroids have beneficial or harmful actions, and I will explain these to you fully.

I will also discuss anabolic steroids later in this chapter so that you will learn how they resemble and differ from other steroids.

Steroids affect the functioning of the body through a chain of events that begins when they attach to complex proteins within the cell. These are called receptors; a hormone has to attach to its special receptor in order to affect the cell. For example, estrogen receptors are present in the quiescent tissue of the breast of a little girl. At puberty, the ovaries make more estrogen, which reaches the breasts through the blood. In the breast, the estrogen attaches to the receptor that activates the genetic potential for the breast to grow. Abnormal events can also be triggered by a hormone attaching to a receptor. For example, androgens can attach to receptors in the hair follicles in the skin of a woman's face and cause hair to grow thicker and darker.

Female Hormones: The Estrogens

The term "female hormone" is a vague one because several different hormones are important in women's bodies. Nonetheless, it is a useful one because it refers to those hormones involved in the special aspects of body function unique to women. The first of the two classes of hormones usually referred to by this term are the estrogens. These feminize the body; in endocrinology, feminization refers to the changes in body shape and in the reproductive organs that occur at puberty: growth of the breasts, widening of the hips, thighs, and buttocks, thickening of the mucosa inside the vagina with an increase in its production of mucus, and the thickening of the lining of the womb, which is shed in menstruation.

There are three major forms of estrogen: estrone, estradiol, and estriol. They differ in two ways: in their chemistry and in the stage of a woman's life they are associated with. The chemi-

Figure 1.

The Ovaries, Adrenals and Their Hormones

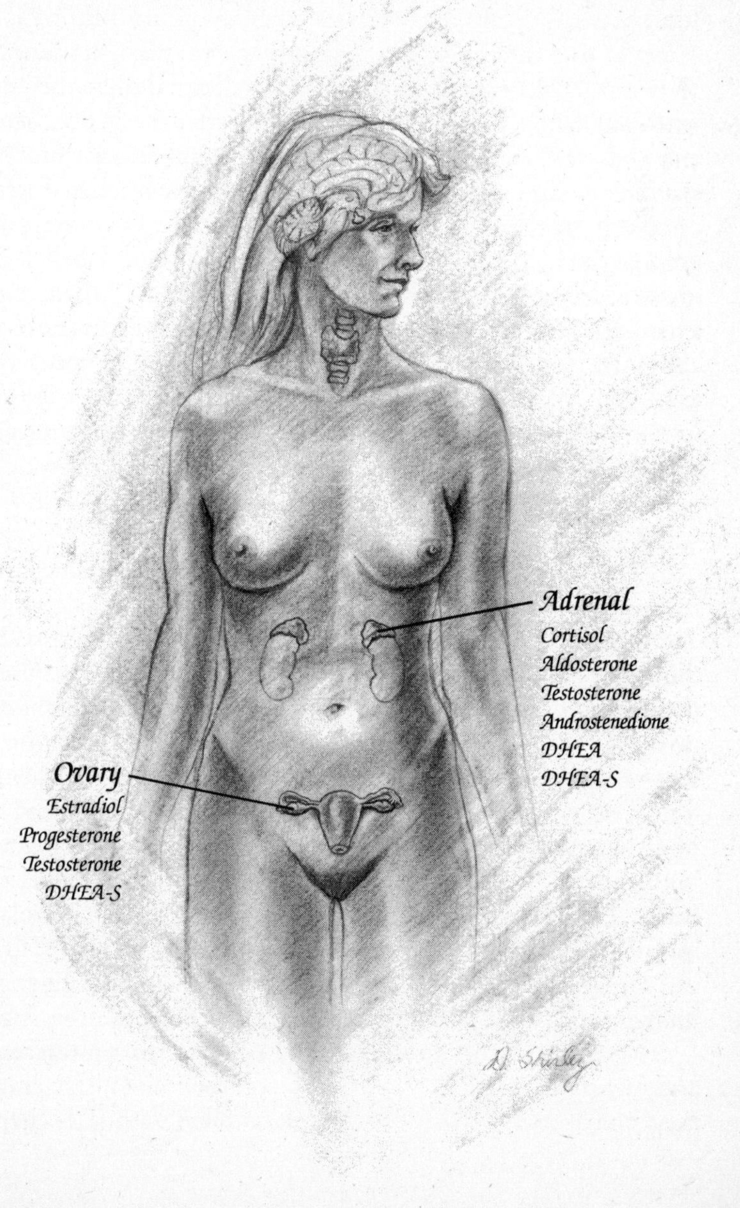

Adrenal
Cortisol
Aldosterone
Testosterone
Androstenedione
DHEA
DHEA-S

Ovary
Estradiol
Progesterone
Testosterone
DHEA-S

cal difference has to do with the number of chemical entities called hydroxyl groups on each hormone molecule. Estrone has one such group; estradiol has two, and estriol three. Each is made in a different place: estrone in fat tissue, estradiol in the ovary, and estriol in the placenta. Estradiol is the main estrogen when the ovary is active, that is, from puberty to menopause. Estriol is high during pregnancy, and estrone predominates after menopause, when the ovary has become quiescent and fat tissue becomes the main source of estrogen. For a long time, researchers were preoccupied with a belief that these estrogens had different effects because of their slight chemical differences. We now know that the effectiveness and safety of estrogen treatment depends not so much on which estrogen you take, but on how it is used.

Although estrogen acts on the brain—for example, in regulating the menstrual cycle—estrogen does not seem to be responsible for sexual feelings in women. The situation in animals is different; estrogen is what causes most female mammals to go into heat. Indeed the word "estrogen" comes from a Greek word meaning "mad with desire." The male animal in turn is aroused by the scent produced by estrogen. While estrogen does not directly induce sexual feeling or behavior in women, it does prepare the vagina to be able to accommodate intercourse. The vagina needs estrogen to function normally. In the absence of estrogen, the wall of the vagina is extremely thin. When estrogen levels rise, as they do in puberty, the mucosal wall becomes thicker, and more mucous is made as lubrication. Every adolescent girl is aware of the increase in vaginal discharge, and many are bothered by it. A related problem in women who are estrogen-deficient is lack of lubrication, as well as thinness of the wall of the vagina, which may make intercourse painful. It is rare, however, for the vagina in an estrogen-deficient woman to be torn during intercourse.

Progesterone and the Progestins

The second kind of female hormone is progesterone. This hormone's effects are termed "pro-gestational" because they prepare a woman's body for gestation, or pregnancy.

Another term, "progestins," refers to the entire class of hormones that can have the biological effects considered progestational. Many of these, such as the progestins used in the birth control pill, are synthetic. While, strictly speaking, progesterone is itself a progestin, more often the term is used to refer specifically to synthetic forms.

Progestins produce effects that cannot be seen, although some can be felt. First is a series of changes in the microscopic appearance of the lining of the uterus (the endometrium). These are called secretory changes, and they are necessary for the endometrium to be able to support a pregnancy if conception has occurred. The secretory changes induced by progesterone include the formation of muscle cells around the capillaries, which can clamp down when menstruation occurs in order to limit blood loss. Without progesterone, periods may be heavy or prolonged. Lack of progesterone also increases cancer risk in the long term, because the endometrial cells do not progress to their proper mature form. Use of progestins to prevent this form of cancer is fully explained in Chapter Thirteen.

Progesterone has widespread effects elsewhere on the body to prepare it for pregnancy. These are familiar to all women because they are experienced in the second half of the menstrual cycle. Fluid retention occurs in order to increase blood volume, since the mother's blood must provide food and oxygen for two. Weight gain provides a store of nutrition for the fetus, and there is stimulation of the breast, producing an increase in size and often a degree of tenderness. Because progesterone also acts on the brain, changes in mood are often experienced during the later part of the cycle.

It is such effects of hormones that give them their mixed reputation. Some unwanted effects are those of natural hormones, while others are effects of hormones taken as medication—birth control pills, estrogen replacement, etc. These medication side effects may be exaggerated forms of normal actions of hormones produced by the body, or they may be novel effects introduced by artificial forms of the hormones.

As a hormone, progesterone can at best be given mixed reviews. It is necessary for preparing the uterus for pregnancy; none of us would be here if it were not for progesterone. Its presence is necessary to protect against cancer of the lining of the uterus. Yet it seems to induce the uncomfortable changes of the late days of the menstrual cycle. There has been what might be described as a "cult" of progesterone. Its leader was Katharina Dalton, a gynecologist in England made famous for her advocacy of the reality of the premenstrual syndrome (PMS). Doctor Dalton's idea was that PMS is the result of too little progesterone in the week before menstruation. We will return to this in Chapter Nine. Here I will simply say that progesterone is the most controversial of the female hormones. Whether it makes women feel better or feel worse is still being debated.

Beyond Male and Female Hormones

In this discussion, we have taken for granted the concept that estrogen and progesterone are "female" hormones. But is this really the right way to look at it? These concepts are more than one hundred years old, dating from a time when female and male were conceived of as absolute opposites. In an age when androgyny is no longer shocking, the assumption that there are distinct male and female hormones can be reexamined. While the concept of female and male hormones is useful as a first approximation, nature is really more subtle than this.

To begin with, progesterone, although a female hormone, is actually the chemical from which *all* other steroid hormones are made. The other "female" hormone, estrogen, and the "male" hormones are made from progesterone. To be sure, the levels of progesterone in the blood of women during the second half of the menstrual cycle are far higher than ever occur in men. But neither men or women can live without progesterone as a source of other hormones.

The most "female" hormone, estrogen, is also present in men and is actually made in the testicle, just as the "male" hormone testosterone is made in women's ovaries. Some men, especially if they are obese, have higher levels of estrogen than occur in normal women during the menstrual phase of their cycle. A small amount of breast tissue is commonly present on a man's body as a result of the action of this estrogen.

Testosterone and other androgens even play an essential role in normal female pubertal development in that they stimulate the appearance of pubic hair. This is why I have used the term "androgens" in this book rather than "male hormones." Androgens belong in a woman's body as much as in a man's, though when levels become high they can cause problems. Having androgens, even when the levels are increased, does not make a woman less feminine, nor does the presence of estrogens in men make us less masculine.

Androgens

Androgens are the forgotten hormones in a woman's body, only thought of when they cause a problem, which unfortunately they often do. Females do not develop as they do because they have no testosterone, but because they have less testosterone. This at first seems to contradict common sense, which regards males and females as completely different. In fact, men and women have more similarities than differences,

Figure 2.

Where Estrogen Acts on a Woman's Body

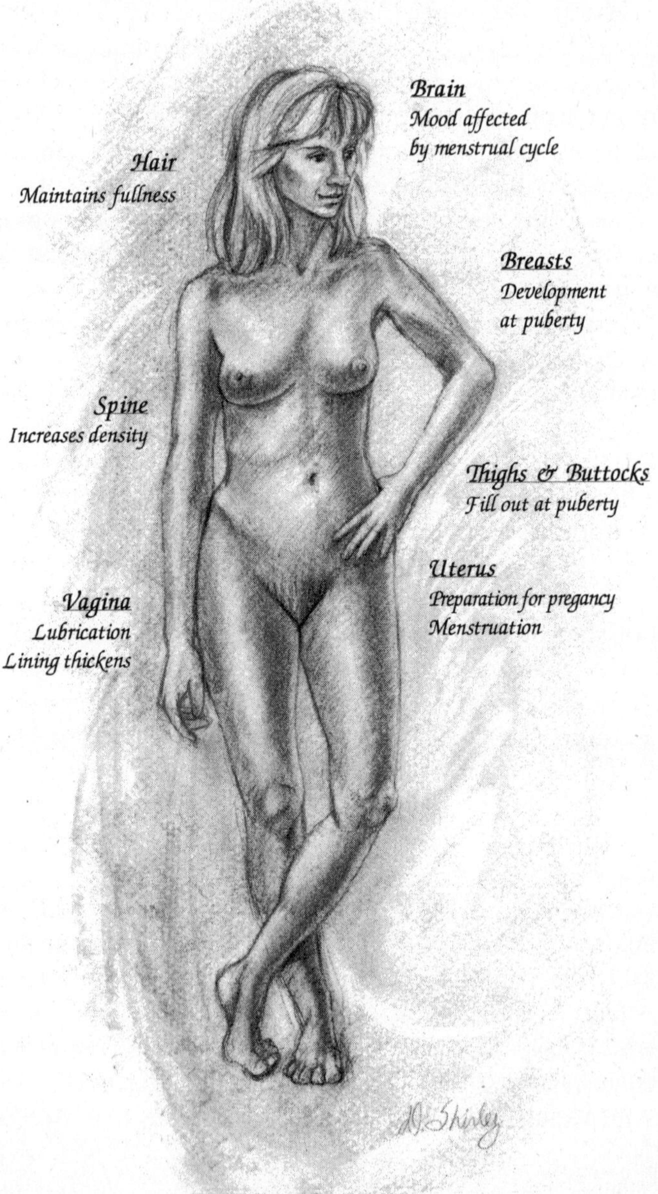

Brain
Mood affected
by menstrual cycle
Hair
Maintains fullness
Breasts
Development
at puberty
Spine
Increases density
Thighs & Buttocks
Fill out at puberty
Uterus
Preparation for pregancy
Menstruation
Vagina
Lubrication
Lining thickens
D. Shirley

but both culture and biology put great emphasis on these differences.

Women vary more than men in their androgen levels. Men, unless they have a disease, have testosterone levels about ten times higher than those in women. These high levels produce near maximal effects on the man's body. Even much higher levels will not produce any more body hair, deeper voice or other masculinizing changes. (The same is true of estrogen levels in healthy menstruating women.) But androgen levels in women are much lower. For women, a small change in androgen level can produce a big change in effect, such as an increase in acne or facial hair growth. Differences in androgen levels in women have more biological significance than they do in men.

While an increase in testosterone can affect a woman's skin and her metabolism, it does not seem to alter mind or behavior. Although testosterone plays some role in libido, few women with increases in testosterone notice anything different in this respect. Some of the women I see for androgen excess report an extremely strong sex drive. Others tell me they have almost no sex drive. Most are in the middle. Males also vary in their sex drive, but this is quite clearly not due to differences in testosterone levels. The most important sex organ is the brain, and it is here that such differences probably reside.

It is only in high school biology that women have no androgens and men no estrogens. However even when high, androgens in women never overlap the male range unless serious disease is present. The average testosterone level in a woman is about 40 ng/dl (nanograms per deciliter; see the section below, on the reporting of hormone test results, for a full explanation) in comparison to 400 ng/dl or higher for a man. A high level for a woman would be 120 ng/dl. So the woman who is told she has "too many male hormones" is far from having levels comparable to a man's.

At various times in medical history, there have been theories that androgens are good for women. For example, there recently has been interest in prescribing a combination of estrogen and the androgen called methyl testosterone for women in menopause who report decreased libido. There are studies suggesting that some women may feel better on this preparation and have a return of sexual desire. However, in premenopausal women, giving testosterone does not increase sexual interest. There is reason to be concerned about the safety of women taking androgens. The problems androgens can cause for women are explained in Chapter Five.

If you have a problem with your sexual desire being less than you think it should be, there are several excellent books that discuss such matters. Lack of interest in sex is almost never due to hormones, with one important exception. Women who feel terrible because they have hormonal conditions that are not being properly treated may not feel sexy simply because they do not feel well. This is not unusual after menopause, because estrogen deficiency makes the whole body feel uncomfortable, as well as weakening the lining of the vagina. If you are having these kinds of problems something can definitely be done (see Chapter Thirteen).

As we have seen, androgens are the hormones responsible for male development, but they are involved in women's development as well. Nature tends to be parsimonious; she uses the same hormones in both sexes. With this in mind, let's look at androgens more closely. Androgens are necessary for a male fetus to develop as a male, and they cause secondary male development at puberty. This includes the male pubertal changes: enlargement of the penis, appearance of pubic, facial, and body hair, oily skin, deepening of the voice, and bulking up of muscle. Increase in muscle size is due to the anabolic effect of androgens, anabolism being the stimulation of the formation of new tissue. (Its opposite is catabolism, which is the breakdown of existing tissue in order to produce energy.)

In males, the anabolic effects of testosterone are necessary for pubertal development. It is less clear what importance androgens have in female development. Androgens do cause the appearance of pubic hair, as well as underarm, facial and body hair. And they make the skin oilier. (These changes and the problems associated with them are discussed in full detail in the chapters on androgenic disorders.) Girls undergo anabolic changes at puberty; their muscles and bones get bigger, though the increase is less dramatic than in boys. There is probably a need for some androgen in female puberty, but not very much. Some girls with increased levels of androgens grow larger than would have been expected, but most adolescent girls with high androgens are normal in size and not necessarily especially muscular.

The Androgens: Some Biochemistry

The most powerful androgen in the body is testosterone. The name means "steroid found in the testes" and that is where the highest concentrations are located. However, testosterone is also produced in women's ovaries and in the adrenal glands of both sexes.

One of the classic controversies of endocrinology has been whether the ovary or adrenal gland is the major source of testosterone in women. Where your body makes most of its testosterone is an individual trait.

It will be useful to you to have at least heard the names of the main androgens, because they are measured when a woman is tested for an androgenic disorder. The minimum you need to know about them in order to understand female androgenic disorders is that there are several important ones (see below) and that when they are too high an androgenic disorder results. Measuring the androgens clarifies the cause of the androgenic disorder and makes it possible to pick the treatment most likely to be effective. If that is all you want to know, you can read just the names of all the androgens in next paragraph so that they are familiar to you and then skip to the next section.

In addition to testosterone, the major androgens are dihydrotestosterone (DHT), androstenedione (or ANDRO), and dehydroepiandrosterone (DHEA) and its sulfate form (DHEA-S). ANDRO is made in the ovary and adrenal glands, just as is testosterone. My research suggests that the ovary is more likely to be the source of ANDRO, but it can be made in both. ANDRO itself is not very active as a hormone, but there is quite a lot of it around. This makes it important because it can be converted chemically either to estrogen or to testosterone. This chemical change of ANDRO to estrogen is one source of estrogen after menopause. DHEA and its similar form DHEA-S come almost entirely from the adrenal glands. DHEA-S is the form that dissolves most easily in the blood, and so there is more of it. Neither seems to act as an androgen, but both can be converted in the body to ANDRO and then these in turn are converted to estrogen or testosterone.

Testosterone is the most important androgen to measure because it is the most active one and is usually the cause of unwanted changes, such as increased facial hair. Why then bother with ANDRO and DHEA-S, since they are not very active? The reason relates to what I have already told you about these compounds. Present in large amounts, they are a source for the body to make testosterone. So if you have excessive levels of either, it may be that your body uses it to make extra testosterone, even though at one particular moment your testosterone level may be normal.

How Are Hormone Test Results Reported?

To understand laboratory test reports you need to know something about units and normal ranges. Test results consist of a number and a unit. The unit is the amount of hormone in a certain volume of serum, the liquid part of blood remaining after it clots. For example, testosterone is usually reported as ng (nanograms or billionths of a gram) contained in each dl (deciliter or 100 ml; equal to a little more than 3 ounces). Hormones are very powerful in their effects on the body, and the amounts that circulate in the blood are exceedingly minute. Estradiol is the most potent, and so levels in the blood are measured in pg (picograms or trillionths of a gram) per ml. (There are 5 ml in 1 teaspoon.)

Unfortunately, not all laboratories use the same units. An estradiol of 50 pg/ml, for example, is the same as 5.0 ng/dl, and a DHEA-S of 300 mcg/dl is the same as 3 ng/ml. If you know how to do metric conversions this should not be a problem. The easier and more enlightening thing to do is to simply look at the normal ranges printed on the lab report. These are very helpful, but remember that they are averages and do not fit all situations. A value just above or below the normal range may or may not really be abnormal. Normal ranges are extremely helpful, but other information often must be taken into account to interpret them. The situation with testosterone is an example. The usual lab normals are set too high. Many labs give their range as up to 70, 80, or even 120 ng/dl, but women who have levels of 50 or higher often notice androgenic changes on their skin or hair.

More About Androgens

Testosterone—like most hormones, including the estrogens— is not simply dissolved in the blood but travels in the circulation attached to a special protein called sex-steroid or sex-hormone binding globulin (SHBG). Most of the testosterone is attached to SHBG, which tends to hold it in the blood and keep it from moving out into the tissues, where it can act. A small amount is dissolved in the blood and is free to move out into these tissues; this is called free testosterone. Free testosterone can be measured and is a much more helpful test than measuring only total testosterone.

Earlier I mentioned one other hormone, DHT or dihydrotestosterone, which is derived from testosterone. An enzyme called 5 alpha reductase converts testosterone to DHT. Conversion of testosterone to DHT in the hair follicle itself seems to increase the effect of testosterone. One theory is that women who have problems with increased hair growth have more of the enzyme 5 alpha reductase and so make more DHT in their hair follicles. There is even a blood test called 3 alpha diol G that is supposed to measure 5 alpha reductase activity. The vogue for this test seems to have waned (some lab tests go in and out of fashion, although doctors and laboratories may not always be willing to admit it). Although I tried this test when it first appeared, it has not turned out to be very helpful. It merely shows what is already obvious: Women with excessive hair have more hormonal activity in their hair follicles. It does not help in figuring out what treatment will work best.

If there is a question of having an androgenic disorder, the most thorough workup will measure total testosterone, free testosterone, androstenedione (ANDRO), and DHEA-S. Levels of DHEA-S in the blood are more steady than levels of DHEA, so it is a more useful measurement. Of these, ANDRO is least important but still useful, especially if you have other signs that you may have an underlying hormone problem (for example, if you often miss periods).

Glucocorticoids

The hormones of this family are often referred to collectively as "corticosteroids," or simply "steroids." Because the latter term has come to be associated with anabolic steroids, I have used the less familiar term "glucocorticoids" to avoid misunderstanding. The effects on the body and the side effects of glucocorticoids are quite different from those of anabolic steroids.

Cortisone was the first hormone discovered in the glucocorticoid family, and its name is familiar to almost everyone. Cortisone is not actually active in the body but is converted first to cortisol. Because it is more familiar, the word cortisone is often used when cortisol or one of its chemically modified pharmaceutical relatives is actually meant. The famous (or infamous) "cortisone shot" is never actually cortisone but a synthetic variant.

Glucocorticoids are essential for life. I mention this at the outset because unfortunately this group of hormones have become better known for their ill effects than for their beneficial ones. Glucocorticoids have as their primary function preparing our bodies to withstand stress. Stress is unpleasant, and the effects necessary for our bodies to withstand it tend to be unpleasant. High levels of glucocorticoid can cause a disturbing "wired" feeling. Glucocorticoids tend to shift metabolism to a defensive mode. This means that tissue is broken down so that it will be available as fuel.

Some people have a deficiency of glucocorticoids. This can occur because the adrenal has been destroyed (usually by the immune system) or because the pituitary is damaged and unable to make the hormone ACTH (adrenocorticotropin), which signals the adrenal to make glucocorticoid. Without ACTH coming from the pituitary, the adrenal will not make adequate amounts of cortisol. When this happens, the body is weak, and the affected person often loses weight. Often these effects are blamed on psychological factors until the diagnosis is made, often by accident. To be fair, Addison's disease (the destruction of the adrenal gland) is very rare, and most people who have problems with their energy level do not have anything wrong with their adrenal gland. When the diagnosis is made and proper medication is taken, energy is restored to normal. In the deficient state, however, people with Addison's disease have great difficulty meeting the demands of job, school, or other responsibilities. Many manage to keep up with their activities by sheer willpower until a physical stress causes them to become acutely ill. Fever, vomiting, or surgery with general anesthesia are hazardous in someone with a lack of glucocorticoids.

For nearly all of us, however, the adrenal gland, under the control of the pituitary gland, can respond to the needs of physical stress, and we are never aware of what would have happened if our adrenal gland were not working. I have stressed that problems with glucocorticoids are rare. They are not particularly female hormone problems but affect both men and women. They can be treated with cortisol or a longer-acting synthetic variant.

Another family of steroids is called mineralocorticoids; they help regulate the balance of the minerals sodium, potassium, and chloride. Aldosterone is the main mineralocorticoid, but it is so rare for women to have problems with it that I have not discussed it in this book.

Pituitary Hormones

The pituitary gland controls many functions in the body, including growth, pubertal development, fertility, and breast milk production. Through its action on the thyroid, it regulates metabolism, and by stimulating the adrenal it makes the body able to withstand stress. Fascinating as the pituitary is, I do not discuss it much in this book because it exerts its effects indirectly on the reproductive system through its actions on other glands. In the interest of clarity, I have given most of my attention to the glands that the pituitary influences, rather than to the pituitary gland itself.

I have included a diagram (page 46) that shows the relationships between the pituitary and the glands it controls.

The pituitary hormones are all small proteins, which are called peptides. This means that chemically they are quite different from the various families of steroids. Their way of acting on the body is also different, because they attach mostly to receptors at the surface of the cell rather than in its interior, as steroids do. Peptides are used as medications, but less often than steroids. One reason is that peptides, like other proteins, are broken down in the stomach and so are not active if given by mouth. Most peptide hormones must be given by injection, although some can be absorbed through the nose. For the pituitary hormones we will be concerned with in this book—growth hormone, luteinizing hormone (LH), and follicle-stimulating hormone (FSH)—injection is still necessary.

As its name suggests, growth hormone is used for stimulating growth in children with severely short stature. It is discussed more fully in the next chapter. LH and FSH are mainly used to induce ovulation in women with infertility due to lack of ovulation. They can help restore sperm production in men who have low counts due to lack of these hormones. The preparations include Pergonal® (Serono), Metrodin® (Serono), and various preparations of human chorionic gonadotropin (hCG), which comes from the placenta and is much like LH. Because this book does not try to cover infertility, I will not discuss the medical preparations of these hormones any further, though I do discuss how FSH and LH regulate female development and the menstrual cycle in the next two chapters.

Figure 3.

The Pituitary and Its Relationship with Other Glands

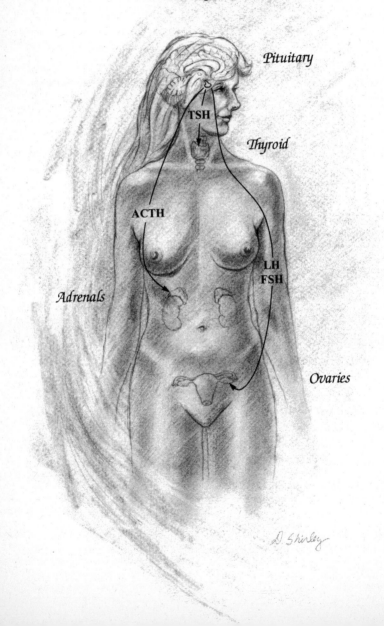

Pituitary

TSH

Thyroid

ACTH

LH
FSH

Adrenals

Ovaries

D. Shirley

Prostaglandins and Menstrual Cramps

Prostaglandins are a family of chemically closely related hormones that are formed in many tissues in the body. They were originally discovered in the prostate gland of men, hence their name. In general, prostaglandins are involved in controlling contraction of the smooth muscle of internal organs, such as that of the blood vessels and airway, as well as the uterus. Ordinary menstrual cramps are the result of excessive production of certain prostaglandins, which cause the uterus to contract painfully. Prostaglandins are also involved in labor and childbirth. A major and familiar class of drugs, the nonsteroidal anti-inflammatory drugs (NSAIDs), work by inhibiting prostaglandin production. These include ibuprofen (Motrin®, Upjohn; Advil®, Whitehall; and Nuprin®, Bristol-Myers). Others are mefenamic acid (Ponstel®, Parke-Davis), naproxin (Naprosyn®, Syntex), sulindac (Clinoril®, Merck), and oxaprozin (Daypro®, Searle). There are many others. Ibuprofen is available without prescription. Pharmaceutical companies promote their NSAIDs heavily, but differences between them are usually small. The important thing to know about NSAIDs is that they work better if taken early so they can prevent the tissues from making the prostaglandins that cause the pain. If you have cramps before or during most of your periods, it is best to start the medication a day or two before you expect cramps to begin and continue for a day longer than you usually have them, since sometimes cramps will last longer than expected. The longer-acting NSAIDs (like sulindac, 500 mg, twice daily, or oxapram, 1,200 mg, once daily) work best because the short-acting ones, such as ibuprofen, start to wear off too quickly, allowing more prostaglandins to form and starting the pain again. On the other hand, for a short-term problem like a headache, ibuprofen is fine in a dose of 400 mg or 600 mg every four hours for a few doses.

The main side effect of NSAIDs is stomach irritation, but

this is mainly a problem in chronic conditions such as arthritis, when large doses must be taken every day. Also, NSAIDs may make asthma worse.

Hormones and Laboratories

The word "test" tends to make everyone uneasy as some are uncomfortable or embarrassing. In endocrinology, most questions can be answered by tests measuring the levels of the hormones themselves in the blood. Each test usually requires only a few ml (milliliters) of blood. The tubes of blood that seem to contain so much of this vital fluid actually hold only 1½ to 2 teaspoons each. Even a big blood draw of ten tubes amounts to only a little more than 3 ounces.

Tests have become so important a part of medicine that one must know something about them to be an adequately informed health-care consumer. Doctors need to know about how the tests they order are done, too, but the great complexity of current clinical medicine leaves less time for training in laboratory science. Yet the laboratory is of ever-increasing importance in medicine, both for diagnosis and for monitoring treatment. There is no complete solution for this. What I can do is explain the pitfalls of laboratory measurements. Laboratories, like other human undertakings, are fallible. In medicine, there recently has been an unfortunate tendency to play down clinical perception—hearing the patient's story, looking at her skin, feeling the thyroid gland or ovary, listening to her heart— as old-fashioned, and to elevate test results to a position of unquestioned authority. Medicine that relies only on tests is bad medicine. Both traditional physical examination and modern testing are necessary.

Like doctors, not all laboratories are the same. Competition brings a wide choice of laboratories and an incentive to introduce new tests that may be very useful in diagnosis. But there is a down side, too. Some laboratories compete on the basis of price by running very large quantities of tests with rather limited quality control. Most results may be right, but some are not, and if it is your result that is wrong, the situation is not helped by the fact that the overall percentage of wrong results is low. Sometimes a disease is missed altogether, and other times the error results in a whole series of other tests that later turn out to have been wholly unnecessary. The cost of these unnecessary tests cannot be recovered, time is lost, and many anxious days are spent. I wish I could say that the situation is improving, but this is not the case. Current pressures for cost containment give the advantage to laboratories that cut costs to the last penny.

Even the best laboratory is not perfect and will have an occasional inaccurate result. I tend to judge a laboratory in large part by how they respond when I question a result. This is something I do whenever the reported finding in the laboratory does not seem to fit the patient's situation. A good laboratory will admit at once the possibility that their test may have developed problems and wants to know right away if something has gone wrong. They will rerun the test at no charge, and even do another test on an additional blood sample, again without charge. In a laboratory that takes its work seriously, I can speak to the chief technician or clinical chemist in charge of that procedure. He or she will call me back when the rerun is completed and tell me exactly what has happened. This is the ideal, and some laboratories operate this way.

Others respond differently. The voice at the other end tells me that there is no problem, there never has been, all their results are 100 percent accurate 100 percent of the time. Laboratories are run by humans, and no humans attain that degree of perfection. Unfortunately the economics of laboratory medicine act to make such responses almost the rule rather than the exception.

Smaller hospital labs mainly act as processing centers; for

all but the most common tests, they simply prepare the blood and send it out to commercial labs for analysis. The problem with this system is that the hospital lab chooses the lab that will do the tests but is not involved in the interpretation of results. They merely reprint them on their own lab report forms and send them on to the doctor who ordered them. Sometimes the report sheet will state the name of the laboratory that actually did the test, but other times it will not. So the patient—and even the doctor—often has no idea where the test was done.

However, there are specialized laboratories in the United States that do excellent work of high accuracy and that stand behind their results. The laboratory I use for my specialized hormonal tests is Endocrine Sciences in Calabasas Hills, California, just north of Los Angeles. This is one of the best laboratories for hormone measurements in the United States and presumably the world. They made their reputation in the most difficult area—doing hormone measurements in children—and so they are usually the first choice of pediatric endocrinologists. Nichols Institute, also in California, is also excellent.

Many large medical schools and other major centers, such as the Cleveland Clinic, the Mayo Clinic, and New York City's Columbia-Presbyterian Medical Center, have excellent laboratories. Yet most institutions, even the most famous, seem to have at least one test they cannot do accurately, and most have several. And even the big medical institutions send some work out to the large commercial labs.

Which tests are hardest to do and require a special lab? Free testosterone is one and TSH another. TSH is thyroid stimulating hormone, the pituitary hormone which controls the thyroid. Very accurate measurement of TSH is important because decisions as to whether to institute lifelong therapy may be made on the basis of very small differences in levels of the hormone. Levels of estrogen and androgens in children and youth are quite low, and below the capabilities of all but a few laboratories. On the other hand, levels of these sex steroids in adults are easy to measure and not much of a problem except at the low end of the range.

Variations in Hormone Levels

There are reasons other than lab errors for test results that seem confusing and inconsistent. The most important is that hormone levels are by no means constant in the blood. Most hormones we want to measure in the blood are not in a steady state. Their levels are dynamic, varying greatly in a variety of patterns. This is because in order for them to regulate body functions, hormone levels have to change in response to different situations. One of the most common patterns of change in hormones is diurnal, or day-night, cycles. Testosterone, for example, is lower in the daytime (especially in the afternoon, when blood is most likely to be drawn after a physical), and so an upper-normal-limit daytime result may suggest a higher than normal level at night. Testosterone and many other hormones also have more or less random short-term fluctuations. This means that a single measurement might give a misleading impression of what the overall levels are. A very evident source of variation in hormone levels is the menstrual cycle itself. In fact, estradiol levels fluctuate so much that it is rarely useful to measure them except in connection with ovulation-induction treatments or to detect menopause. The possibility of fluctuations must be considered by the doctor in interpreting the tests.

Hormones as Medications

In endocrinology, hormones have two aspects: as chemicals made in the body and as chemicals we place in our bodies in the form of medication. In most ways, hormones taken as medication act similarly to the natural hormones; that is why they are taken. But there can be differences, and these need to be understood by you and by your doctor. In some cases, the differences are deliberate, making the hormone more suitable or convenient when taken as a drug. Other differences are unwanted but unavoidable, because the natural hormone cannot be made or cannot be absorbed into the body in its natural form, or would not last long enough if it did.

An easy way to understand this is to consider what has to happen for a hormone to be an effective medication. First, the structure of the hormone has to be known and a method for making it discovered. After the structure of the hormone is known, a method to manufacture it must be invented. This was accomplished in the 1950s and 1960s for steroids, and in the 1980s for peptides, which now are made with recombinant DNA technology. The ability to inexpensively synthesize estrogens and progestins was the breakthrough that permitted practical oral contraception. What is produced outside the body is referred to as synthetic. To a pharmacologist, a synthetic drug is often better because it is usually purer, as well as cheaper to produce. And as much can be made as is needed. I'll return to the issue of natural versus synthetic shortly.

After the hormone has been made, it must be formulated— that is, put into a form suitable for storage and eventual introduction into the body. Once in the body, the hormone must be absorbed. In the case of an oral medication, it must leave the stomach intact after exposure to the hydrochloric acid there. And in the small intestine it must escape destruction by digestive enzymes. It also must dissolve in water; otherwise, it cannot pass from the liquid intestinal contents into the bloodstream.

Nor are the problems over when the medication is safely into the bloodstream. From the intestine, blood flows directly through the liver, which chemically inactivates many substances absorbed from food that might otherwise have unwanted effects on body function. This action of the liver to remove drugs and other substances from what is absorbed from the intestine is called the first-pass effect, and certain hormones are not effective when given by mouth because the liver destroys them. There are two ways around this problem. One is to give the hormone by injection so that the liver is bypassed. The other solution is for a new molecule to be designed that will be resistant to being broken down by the liver. Obviously this is not easy to do. Synthetic hormones can differ from natural ones only within definite limits. If a hormone-like molecule differs too much from the natural hormone, it will not affect the body at all.

After all this, the hormone must then act on its target tissue. Usually this requires it be present in the blood for a prolonged period of time, from several hours to several days. Most hormones, however, are broken down within a few minutes. This means that many of the hormones used as drugs have been altered so that they stay in the blood for a longer time. An example is ethinyl estradiol, the form of estrogen used in low-dose birth control pills. Ethinyl estradiol is estrogen modified in a way that makes it last hours in the blood instead of minutes. Without this alteration, the contraceptive pill would have to be taken many times a day for it to be reliable.

Some hormones, such as insulin and growth hormone, must be given by injection. Testosterone also is usually given by injection. No one likes the idea of injections, but most people find that if they need them regularly they get used to them more easily than they imagined. Nowadays people are taught to give themselves injections if they will be required more than occasionally. Although many fear that they will not be able to learn, I have never known anyone who could not do so when there was good reason. It is my consistent observation that women can learn to give themselves injections far more easily than men.

Natural and Synthetic Hormones

The label "natural" immediately gives rise to a favorable feeling. And "synthetic" seems suspect, possibly harmful, in any event not as good as the natural version. The truth is more complex. There are two kinds of distinction between natural and synthetic. The first is the difference between something prepared from a substance found in nature and something manufactured. The second is the difference between substances that are normally present in the body and substances that would never be there if they were not taken as medications. A more precise term than "natural" for substances normally found in the body is "native." In contrast to other forms of medication, hormones are more likely to be native or very similar to native substances.

Many people assume that natural substances are inherently safer than synthetic ones. However, there are important exceptions to this principle. Not all man-made chemicals are harmful, and not all natural ones are safe. Human growth hormone is one such example. For nearly three decades after its introduction in 1957 it could be obtained only by extracting it from the pituitaries of cadavers obtained at autopsies. In those early days, it was available to treat children with a form of extremely short stature due to deficiency of the hormone. More recently, the hormone has been made synthetically through recombinant DNA technology. As this new form was nearing completion of testing prior to being approved by the FDA, it was discovered that a virus causing a rare brain disease, Jacob-Creutzfeld's disease, may have been present in the natural growth hormone preparations. Fortunately only a very few cases occurred. Natural does not necessarily mean safe. The currently used growth hormone preparations made with recombinant DNA have never had any problems with infection.

Because of the confusion surrounding the use of the terms "natural" and "synthetic," I will try to avoid them as much as possible in this book. Please do not think, however, that just because I don't always think "natural" is better that I think what a woman puts in her body is unimportant. The only way to be confident that a substance is safe is for it to have been carefully tested. I will discuss safety issues in detail for all the hormones and other medications I discuss. I will also explain how they are related to the natural hormone they are modeled on and what differences in effect synthetic hormones may have.

This leads to one of the most important points I will make in this book and one that will also apply to other medical treatments unrelated to your hormones: Generally drugs in themselves are not safe or dangerous. Rather *it is how they are used that makes them dangerous or safe*. Birth control pills are quite safe in younger women who do not smoke and who are healthy. But in an older woman who smokes and has high blood pressure they may be dangerous. Another example is estrogen therapy after menopause. Used alone or with inadequate progesterone it can cause cancer of the endometrium (the lining of the uterus). But with proper progestin use, the risk of this kind of cancer actually goes down.

I will try to be as specific as possible about how hormones should be used as medications. I will explain both safe and dangerous uses. And I will alert you to warning signs of possible problems. This need not be taken in a negative way. If adverse effects are known and understood, they can be dealt with. Although sometimes they must be lived with, more often they can be prevented, minimized, or counteracted.

Medications are taken in the hope of enhancing health or quality of life. Because of widely publicized mishaps with pharmaceuticals in the past, many women are wary of taking medicines, especially for long-term use. But avoiding medication itself is not necessarily good. Many wish to correct their problem through lifestyle change, diet, vitamins, or other means. Often these things do help. At other times, they may be ineffective or even harmful. While knowledge about health has exploded in the last decades, it is still incomplete. When there is controversy, both sides tend to present their case in extreme language. Since life, health, and fertility are at stake, this does not make decision making easier. There is no simple solution except for women to be as well informed as possible regarding any medication they are considering taking.

Estrogens

Estrogens are very potent chemicals in their effect on a woman's body. For this reason, the body must be able to prevent them from building up in excessive levels; the liver is able to remove estrogen from the blood very quickly. This makes it harder to use estrogens as medications since they tend to be removed almost as quickly as they enter the blood. To add another problem, estrogens do not dissolve well in water and so cannot be easily absorbed from the intestine. Fortunately these problems have been solved in a number of creative ways, and a variety of estrogen preparations are available. This does mean that choices have to be made from among several different forms of estrogen on the basis of data that are sometimes confusing. But it also means that there is usually a way a woman who needs estrogen can take it without major side effects.

(I will mention the main preparations here and then return to this subject in several of the following chapters. My goal in this section is to give you the background information that you need to understand the options in estrogen therapy. I will tell you later what works best in particular situations.)

ESTRADIOL

This is the natural or active estrogen in women from puberty through menopause. Its wide use in the United States is relatively recent, but it has been very widely used in Europe. The brand name is Estrace® (Mead-Johnson).

CONJUGATED ESTROGEN

This form of estrogen, politely termed "conjugated equine estrogen," may seem rather peculiar. The "conjugation" is a straightforward chemical modification that makes estrogen water-soluble and therefore absorbable, and the "equine" refers to the origin of this preparation in horses. Contained in it are two estrogens unique to horses, equilin and equinilan. This preparation is the form of estrogen replacement most widely used in the United States. It has major advantages for some women and for adolescent girls who need hormonal help to go through puberty.

TRANSDERMAL ESTROGEN

This form is the most imaginative and high-tech. The hormone is placed in a special plastic patch that is applied to the skin. Over a period of three days the hormone gradually passes through the skin into the blood. Because it enters the blood at a steady rate, the levels in the blood stay fairly constant. This is a great advantage for those women who are very sensitive to estrogen and experience side effects such as nausea if the levels get even slightly higher than needed. Pills give peaks and valleys: high levels right after the pill is taken and low ones just before the next is due. For most women this variation is not a problem. But for those who are very sensitive to estrogen side effects, transdermal estrogen often works out best.

ETHINYL ESTRADIOL AND MESTRANOL

These are the most commonly used estrogens because they are the ones contained in birth control pills. They are chemically modified by the attachment of what is called an ethinyl group to the estradiol molecule. Mestranol is ethinyl estradiol with an additional chemical group tacked onto it, but because this introduces some variation in the activity of the hormone, it is not used in current, low-dose birth control pills. The invention of ethinyl estradiol was a great advance, one of those that made possible oral contraception.

Progesterone and Progestins

With progesterone the situation is somewhat less satisfactory than with estrogens. A variety of synthetic variants exists, and it is still controversial to what degree these have different effects than progesterone itself. More precisely, the debate is about whether these effects are harmful; there is no doubt that the modified progestins have some effects on the body that do not occur with progesterone itself. We will take this issue up in much more detail in Chapters Twelve and Thirteen. Progesterone derivatives are more distant in their chemical relation to progesterone itself than are estrogen preparations to estradiol.

NATIVE PROGESTERONE

Progesterone is not well absorbed when taken orally. Various ways have been tried to resolve this problem. One, the oldest, is to dissolve progesterone in oil and then give it by intramuscular injection. This causes it to be slowly released over a period of hours or days. It is impractical for long-term use because of the need for several injections each cycle. Progesterone in oil is sometimes used to bring on a period in women who are not menstruating, but this is done less now than formerly. It tends to be used more in emergency rooms than in private doctors' offices.

Many drugs not absorbed from the gastro-intestinal tract can be absorbed across mucous membranes, including those of the lining of the vagina and rectum. Progesterone is sometimes used in suppository form. These can be placed in either the vagina or the rectum. Their main use has been as a way to administer natural progesterone for women with severe PMS. However, most women find suppositories too inconvenient to be an acceptable alternative to tablets.

More recently, micronized progesterone has been made in capsule and tablet form. Micronization is a method of manufacture in which the hormone is divided into tiny microscopic particles that can then dissolve easily to permit absorption. (It is also used for estradiol.) There is less experience with these preparations than with the other progestins, but they do show promise.

MEDROXYPROGESTERONE ACETATE (MPA)

The brand name for this most widely used progestin is Provera®. A newer brand of MPA that may be cheaper is Cycrin® (Wyeth-Ayerst). A closely related drug that is used far less often is megestrol, or Megace® (Mead-Johnson). Megestrol is mainly used in high doses for treatment of endometrial cancer. MPA is commonly used with hormone replacement for menopause and other forms of estrogen deficiency. These progestins are quite close to progesterone in their structure but are more likely to cause mood changes. Some women who take MPA experience premenstrual-like symptoms such as cramps, fluid retention, depression, and weight gain. These usually occur in women who have had a tendency to premenstrual symptoms before they needed hormone replacement. Some, however, clearly feel worse with MPA than with natural periods. One reason may be that commonly used doses are relatively high. In usual doses, MPA does not appear to have unfavorable effects on lipid levels. Since a major reason for giving hormone replacement is to reduce the risk of heart disease, this advantage is a very important one.

The long-acting form of MPA has the brand name Depo-Provera® (Upjohn). When given by injection, it can last several months if the dose is high enough. This has made it useful as an injectable contraceptive, especially in developing countries, in which it may be difficult for women to take birth control pills every day on schedule. During the time DepoProvera is having its effect, there are no full periods, but there may be light but prolonged and unpredictable bleeding. In women with mental retardation, DepoProvera is sometimes used to stop menses or to provide effective contraception. Thus Depo-Provera has been given to women who are not really able to give informed consent to its use. Advocates for these groups have questioned its use on grounds both of safety and of ethics. From a medical point of view, DepoProvera appears to be a very safe drug. However, it has limited usefulness in the treatment of hormonal disorders, and few women who read this book will consider its use.

Another progestin with chemical similarities to MPA is cyproterone acetate (CPA). It is available in most countries under the brand name Androcur® (Schering A.G.). It is not now available in the United States, although it will be soon under some rather special circumstances. What is of interest about CPA is that it is an anti-androgen. This means it blocks the action of the androgen group of hormones; this will be discussed in detail in Chapter Six on the treatment of androgenic disorders.

BIRTH CONTROL PILLS AND THEIR PROGESTINS

Birth control pills use progestins that have some chemical similarities to testosterone, the main androgen or male hormone. Their principal disadvantage is that they have androgenic side effects. Fortunately some pills are much less likely to cause these effects than others. The newest birth control pills have progestins that are virtually free of this problem. (See Chapter Twelve.)

It may be tempting to throw up one's hands at the great variety of hormone preparations available. But remember that one reason for inventing new forms of drugs is not science but business. The reason the pills have various progestins is that different companies wanted a progestin they could patent and then develop into their own line of oral contraceptives. The resulting research was mainly commercial in intent but sometimes led to introduction of better forms of drugs. From the point of view of the woman considering using a progestin, many of the differences are not important. In the later chapters on specific hormone problems, I will tell you which progestins seem best.

Androgens as Medications: Testosterone Replacement

For a woman who feels she has a low sex drive, taking testosterone will not make any difference, though women who have had their ovaries removed may be an exception. Since a woman's body is extremely sensitive to the effects of testosterone, even brief treatment with it may cause increased body and facial hair, which may then require further treatment. Androgens may help in certain rare conditions; some of these are discussed in the following section on anabolic steroids.

Anabolic Steroids

Metabolism has two phases: anabolism, in which tissue is built up, and catabolism, in which it is broken down. Catabolism is necessary for our bodies in certain temporary situations but is harmful over the long term. Aging is a state in which catabolism is relatively predominant over anabolism. The mass of muscle and bone gradually decreases while fat increases. Even if there is no change in body weight, as a man or woman ages, his or her body has increasing amounts of fat and decreases in muscle and bone.

The deleterious effects of catabolism have been recognized for several decades. Some situations cause metabolism to become more catabolic. Aging is one; others are kidney failure, liver disease, congestive heart failure, advanced cancer, and certain blood diseases in which the bone marrow is unable to make enough new blood cells. In these states, anabolism cannot be induced by nutritional means. This led to a search for drugs or hormones that could shift metabolism to the anabolic mode.

In the 1950s, medical scientists thought of trying to use the anabolic properties of testosterone to help patients with these diseases. Testosterone itself might be used to promote anabolism in patients with kidney disease or anemia due to a weakened bone marrow. But it would really only be suitable for men because the other effects of testosterone—increasing body hair, deepening of the voice, receding of the hair line—are disfiguring to women. So researchers sought to separate the anabolic effects of testosterone from the male developmental effects. The result is a group of chemicals derived from testosterone known as anabolic steroids.

Once anabolic steroids were a rather obscure group of drugs used only in a few rare situations. Then someone thought of using them in another situation in which anabolism is important: athletic training. The greater muscle bulk of males is due to their tenfold higher testosterone levels. What if it were increased farther, perhaps another tenfold? Could muscle mass be increased even more? For a long time, medical scientists were skeptical, endocrinologists even more than most. We all believed that testosterone levels in normal men were maximal, that giving more would not make any difference. This belief was incorrect.

Anabolic steroids, if taken in massive doses, do increase anabolism sufficiently that muscle size and strength can be increased beyond what is normally possible. It is hard for most people to see the point of this. For most, sports are a way of improving health and feeling in greater control of our bodies and more harmonious with them. The naturalness of sports activity is one of its greatest appeals. Unfortunately the great emphasis on winning in sports today and the economic rewards of being a superior athlete cause some to use anabolics in the hope of improving their performance.

Women take anabolics, too. Their use is especially common among bodybuilders and in track. Many women who use anabolics develop definite masculinizing changes in their bodies, although they may be photographed in a way that hides these changes. These changes are not entirely reversible, so women who use them pay a big price.

How dangerous are anabolics? There is less scientific information about this than one might think. The synthetic changes in the androgen molecule that make it absorbable by mouth cause it to be potentially toxic to the liver. Two liver problems can result. Peliosis hepatis is a change in the structure of the liver that increases the size of blood vessels in it and thus may make it more vulnerable to injury, such as in a contact sport like football. Tumors can also form within the liver as a result of anabolic steroid use. However, both of these complications are exceedingly rare.

This does not mean that anabolics are safe. Because use of anabolics is secret, it is difficult to gather information about their long-term effects. Because certain of the actions of androgens promote atherosclerosis, there is reason for serious worry about later effects. But the main problems with anabolics are social and ethical. Sports heroes should not use illegal drugs, and their performance should be to their own efforts. Medical use of anabolics is diminishing. For bone marrow problems, especially those related to kidney disease, better treatments have been found. The kidney hormone erythropoietin, made with recombinant DNA, is far more effective in raising the red blood cell count than anabolics.

Medical Use of Glucocorticoids

Many women will have occasion for themselves or someone in their family to take glucocorticoids. Strictly speaking, glucocorticoids are not female hormones, although they are used for treatment of androgenic disorders involving the adrenal gland. If you have no reason to be concerned about this class of hormones, you can skip this section.

Conditions in which the adrenal gland makes too much or too little cortisol are rare. Much more common are problems that come about because of their use as medications. Despite their side effects, which I shall discuss shortly, glucocorticoids (the family of hormonal medications that include cortisol) are essential in modern medicine in virtually all specialties. Their use is related not to the roles in the body that I have described but to their ability to suppress inflammation and the immune response. While the immune system is needed to protect our bodies against infection, all too often it goes into overdrive and in its effort to destroy invading organisms damages normal tissue as well.

The list of diseases for which cortisol or its relatives are effective is a very long one. Some, like rheumatoid arthritis, cause considerable disability and pain. Others, like lupus or asthma, can be fatal. When cortisone was discovered in the 1950s, it seemed like a miracle and was tried for almost everything. That was early in the era of potent drugs, and the potential for side effects was unrecognized. It was not long, however, before the problems of cortisone became apparent.

When glucocorticoids are taken for more than a few days, adverse effects begin to show themselves. The most obvious is that least welcome of hormonal effects, weight gain. Under the influence of cortisol, protein is broken down and converted into sugar and eventually into fat. The fat is distributed on the body in a peculiar way, in which the face and trunk get bigger and rounder while the arms and legs are spared. To make matters worse, the skin is weakened because collagen, the protein that gives skin its strength, has been broken down for conversion to glucose. As the skin is pulled as a result of the weight gain, its weakened condition causes it to thin excessively, and stretch marks result. Ordinary stretch marks are simply due to stretching of the skin either from ordinary weight gain or from other changes in the shape of the body, such as breast development at puberty or the swelling of the abdomen in pregnancy. They usually heal gradually and become almost invisible. The stretch marks resulting from glucocorticoid are worse because the skin has been made thinner by the medication.

The metabolic effects of cortisol are also harmful. Bone

building is inhibited; as a result, calcium is gradually lost since the body is less able to maintain the bones. Fractures can result either from relatively minor injury or, in the case of the spine, from gravity. I have mentioned that cortisol causes protein to be converted into glucose; sometimes the body cannot fully compensate and blood sugar becomes abnormally high, resulting in diabetes.

All this sounds very grim. Fortunately doctors are well aware of these effects and use glucocorticoids very carefully. The side effects are related to dose, but even more to how long a person takes the medication. A course of a few days or even one or two weeks at usual anti-inflammatory doses rarely causes problems. However, some inflammatory conditions are chronic, and for them a short course of therapy is not sufficient. Generally glucocorticoids do not cure conditions but simply suppress them.

There has been great effort to find ways of minimizing the side effects of glucocorticoids. An obvious way is to limit the length of time they are taken, if possible. For many years, the pharmaceutical industry sought ways to modify the cortisol molecule so that the beneficial effects could be preserved but the side effects eliminated. Unfortunately this effort was really successful only to a very limited degree. Many new analogues of cortisol were developed, and some have important advantages, but none are free of side effects.

One successful approach was the development of topical therapy in which cortisol is applied directly to the affected tissue, resulting in high levels where they are needed, but without the rest of the body being exposed to them. This works so well on the skin that use of hydrocortisone or other glucocorticoid skin creams is the most common treatment for skin diseases.

There are also a variety of oral forms of glucocorticoid. The most useful ones are: prednisone (Deltasone®, Upjohn), methylprednisolone (Medrol®, Upjohn), and dexamethasone (Decadron®, Merck). These have three general differences from cortisol. They are more powerful, milligram for milligram, so that a smaller number of milligrams are given. To give approximate equivalences, prednisone is five times as potent as cortisol, and methylprednisolone is about 25 percent more powerful than prednisone. Dexamethasone is ten times more powerful than prednisone, and fifty times more potent than cortisol. Dexamethasone's effects on the body last more than twenty-four hours after a single dose. The long period of action is often an advantage because the medication does not need to be taken as often. However, combined with the drug's great potency, it also means that side effects are more likely unless it is prescribed with extreme care by a physician experienced in this kind of treatment. Care in the use of glucocorticoid drugs is necessary in any case.

There is one remaining difference between these medication forms of glucocorticoid—their salt-retaining activity. The synthetic glucocorticoids I have discussed have much less salt-retaining effect than cortisol and so are preferred in almost all situations. Dexamethasone has the least, and so can even be used in situations such as brain swelling, in which hydrocortisone could make matters worse.

GLUCOCORTICOID DOSES

It will be useful to give some ideas of doses for these glucocorticoids. This subject is often misunderstood, even by physicians. There are two kinds of dosing for all glucocorticoids. The first is called the physiological replacement dose. This is simply the amount equivalent to what the adrenal gland usually makes. "Physiological" here means that the effects are those that happen in the normal functioning of the body. The other is the pharmacological dose, which is larger and has effects on the body that are those of a medication rather than the normal hormonal effects. In general, side effects are a problem only at the higher, pharmacological doses. Since pharmacological doses are used more often, their effects are more familiar to most doctors and their patients.

Children need lower doses, and formulas exist to calculate them. Children experience the same side effects as adults, with another unfortunate one: slowing of their growth. The bone effects that result in calcium loss in adults cause the bones to stop growing in children. Growth hormone can partially overcome this effect.

Physiological doses of glucocorticoids do not have the side effects that the pharmacological doses do. These very safe low doses are the ones most often used to treat endocrine conditions. I emphasize this because the side effects of higher-dose regimens should not deter someone who needs a replacement dose because of a hormonal disorder of the adrenal or pituitary gland. Those who need to take glucocorticoid replacement are those who have an adrenal or a pituitary problem that makes their adrenal gland not able to make enough cortisol. This includes those with the very rare Addison's disease, as well as those who have had pituitary tumors or pituitary underactivity from other conditions.

Low doses of a glucocorticoid can be helpful to some women with androgenic disorders because they suppress adrenal androgen production. However, it is critically important that no more than the physiological dose be used. I have seen women who had been put on doses of dexamethasone that were too high; they experienced weight gain and very bad stretch marks as a result. Some articles and textbooks recommend dexamethasone doses of 0.5 or 0.75 mg daily. I believe these are too high. A few years ago I did a study, published in the *Journal of the American Academy of Dermatology*, of what does of dexamethasone is needed to suppress androgens into the normal range. We found that no woman needed a dose higher than 0.375 mg per day, and most had corrections of their elevated androgen level on 0.125 or 0.25 mg. At these lower doses, no one developed stretch marks, and overall there was no weight gain. If done properly, this treatment is safe so long as the dose is not excessive.

The length of therapy is the most important variable in causing side effects with glucocorticoid. A few days of dexamethasone at a much higher dose will have fewer side effects than a lower (but still pharmacological) dose taken for many months. If you take dexamethasone for a female hormone problem, do not take more than 0.25 mg a day unless that dose has been proved by testing to be ineffective in suppressing your androgens or if you are taking it for a short time to help you conceive.

TAPERING GLUCOCORTICOIDS

Stopping glucocorticoids properly is just as important as taking them correctly. Under some circumstances it is best to reduce the dose slowly. There are two reasons for this. First, the condition being treated may rebound. This doesn't happen with hormonal disorders, but it can happen with some inflammatory conditions such as rheumatoid arthritis or with brain swelling problems. Second, the adrenal suppression I discussed in the previous section may be long-lasting. In this case, it is best if the dose is reduced in slow steps, allowing the adrenal gland to partially recover before the dose is further reduced. If this is not done, the symptoms of underactivity of the adrenal gland, especially fatigue, can occur. (If you have an adrenal problem, you should be under the care of an endocrinologist and certainly not rely simply on the instructions in this or any other book.)

For a woman with normal adrenals who has been on dexamethasone for suppression of androgens, there is no problem with stopping the dexamethasone abruptly, but I usually suggest doing so in several steps of a few months each. One reason for this is that if the androgen-related problem comes back it will not do so in as severe a way, and the dexamethasone dose can be put back to the higher one again.

There is one more thing you should know about stopping glucocorticoid therapy, which also has to do with the fact that the adrenal gland takes many months to completely recover its ability to make cortisol. Remember that the most important role of cortisol is to prepare the body for stress. The body's way of handling such events as fever, vomiting, or general anesthesia depends on the adrenal gland. However, if the adrenal gland is damaged or still suppressed by present or recent glucocorticoid therapy, it does not always have the reserve needed to increase cortisol levels sufficiently. In this case, a supplemental dose may be needed. If you are or have been on any of the glucocorticoid medications I have discussed or one of the other less commonly used ones, you will need a higher dose for any of the situations I have mentioned. You should also make sure your doctor and any close relative whose help would be sought in an emergency knows about it. Sometimes it is a good idea to have a vial of injectable cortisol (hydrocortisone) at home, in case an emergency arises.

The minidoses that I have described for androgenic disorders (0.125 to 0.375 mg of dexamethasone) do not generally suppress the adrenal gland enough to cause it to be unable to respond to stress. None of the women I have treated this way have ever had any difficulty. Nonetheless if you have been on any glucocorticoid and feel unusually ill with flu or vomiting, or if you are having surgery, your doctor should know that you have been on glucocorticoid.

In this chapter I have introduced the main hormones that affect a woman's well-being, described their actions on the body, and briefly explained how they are measured in the laboratory. And I have described the main pharmaceutical preparations of hormones and related medications. In the chapters to come I will put this somewhat theoretical information into practical form and explain how it can be used to help women with actual hormone problems.

Chapter Three

•

How Hormones Shape Female Development from Before Birth Through Puberty and Adulthood

*L*et us return to Tracey, who started to develop breasts at three years of age. Tracey's mother was very anxious about the changes in her daughter's body. She wondered what strange thing could be happening, and how she could face puberty in a three-year-old.

Before dealing with the psychological aspects of the situation, I had to evaluate Tracey's early puberty from a purely medical point of view. Her story was simple. Three or four months earlier, Tracey's mother had noticed what looked like breasts and pointed this out to her own mother. Both thought it might just be weight gain. Then, about a month before the visit to me, her mother noticed a few short, but nonetheless dark and noticeable pubic hairs. She knew this could not be attributed to weight gain. A visit to their pediatrician followed, and she was from there referred to me.

I was relieved to find there were no other symptoms, no behavior suggestive of headaches, no unexplained vomiting. These can be symptoms of a brain tumor, though usually they are not. (Brain tumor headaches usually occur in the morning on awakening and frequently are associated with nausea or vomiting. A little later, the symptoms go away, and so they are often attributed to a wish to avoid school. This morning headache pattern is unusual and must be taken seriously when it occurs.) Nor did Tracey have any vaginal bleeding. This can occur in little girls, although it is rare. It would suggest a problem, possibly even a tumor, in the ovary.

When I examined Tracey, I found just what one would expect to find in a girl just starting puberty—breast buds, some increased curviness of her hips, and a few short but thick, black hairs on the mons veneris, the mound of flesh just above the vagina. These changes would not have caused any concern had Tracey been over eight years old, the youngest normal age for puberty to begin. In this situation, a rectal examination is sometimes done; it permits the ovaries and uterus to be felt, much as a pelvic examination does for an adult woman, but without involving the vagina, which is quite small and delicate in little girls. The next step with Tracy was to do some tests to see what was causing her to go into puberty too early.

I explained to Tracey's mother that precocious puberty is just normal puberty at the wrong time. Puberty is something programmed into all of us; while it usually does not begin until eight or older, it can start at any age. In order to be sure that there was no abnormality of the structure of the pituitary gland or hypothalamus, a magnetic resonance imaging (MRI) scan would be needed. If she'd had more than a slight amount of pubic hair, I would have measured testosterone and DHEA-S also. Tracey's estradiol level was only in the early pubertal range, which reassured me that she did not have an estrogen-producing tumor of the ovary because when that happens the levels are very high. Had it been high, an ultrasound of the ovaries would have been able to show whether she had a tumor there. For the MRI scan, I sent Tracey to a center that has experience with brain tumors in children, because a tumor could be so small on

Figure 4.

Development of Breasts and Pubic Hair:
Tanner Stages

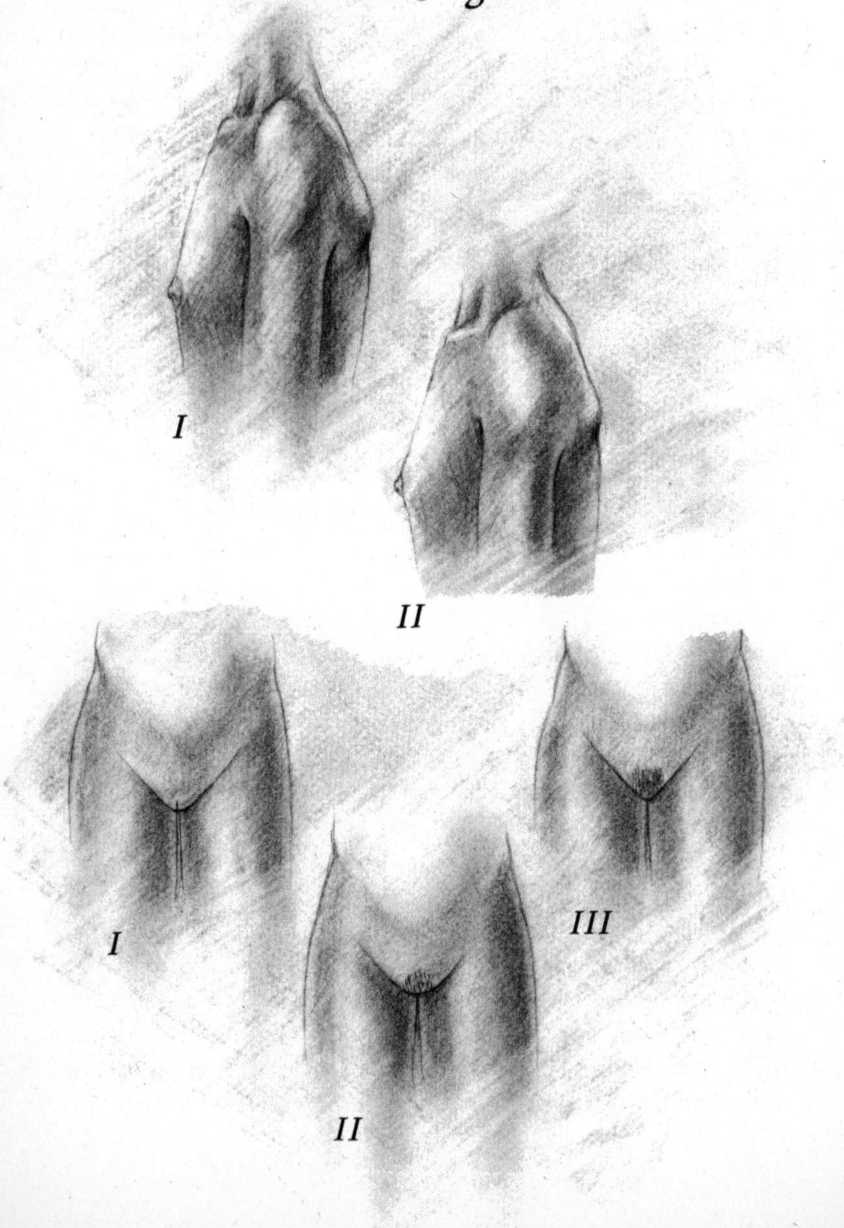

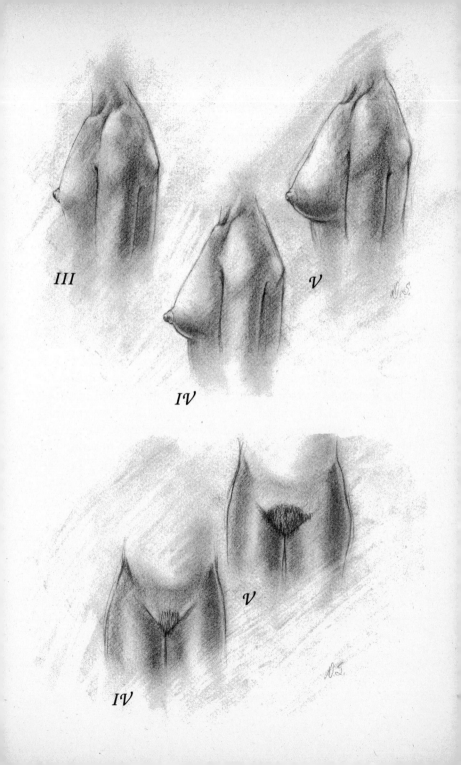

an X ray that neuroradiologists not used to this problem could overlook it.

MRIs are painless, but small children cannot sit still in the machine, which is necessary for a clear picture to be obtained. For this reason, Tracey was given an intravenous injection of a sedative, and she was also given an injection of something called gadolinium, which functions like a dye to make the circulation show up more clearly on the pictures. We were all relieved when Tracey's MRI turned out to be normal.

Tracey's breast development was only late stage II, meaning that she had only small nubbins of tissue under the nipples. I suggested to Tracey's mother that we wait a few months before starting treatment to be certain that her puberty was actually advancing. Occasionally a little girl will start to develop, but then this will stop on its own. If it were going to stop, she would not need medication. On the other hand, if she did advance in puberty, three years old was much too young and Tracey should receive treatment. Her mother agreed to waiting, and indeed seemed relieved, because she was nervous about the long-term effects of hormonal medicine. We agreed that Tracey would come back to see me in three months.

When Tracey came back, her breasts had definitely grown larger. I had used a soft plastic ruler to measure the amount of breast tissue; this made it possible for me to know with certainty that her breast tissue had increased. It was important to find this out because there is a much milder situation called precocious thelarche (thelarche means the start of breast development). In precocious thelarche, there is a slight enlargement of the breast, but no other pubertal changes; the breast soon stops developing, softens, and does not enlarge again until puberty starts at the normal age. Precocious thelarche is a harmless condition that needs no treatment because it is self-limited. It is due to a temporary increase in estrogen production by the little girl's ovary.

I explained to Tracey's mother that a medication called leuprolide would hold off puberty unto the proper age. Tracey remained on leuprolide until she was ten and a half, the average normal age for puberty to begin. Once leuprolide was stopped, her development resumed.

Although boys get precocious puberty far less often than girls, it can happen, and because of behavioral effects may be a more difficult problem. Leuprolide and related medications (Gn-RH analogues) work for boys, too, fortunately. However, there is less complete information on the effects of the treatment on reproduction. In girls, there does not seem to be any unfavorable effect on fertility. As we shall discuss later on in this book, leuprolide is used for several adult female problems; it seems not to interfere with the ability to get pregnant once the drug is discontinued.

I have told Tracey's story to illustrate the nature of pubertal disorders; they are the right things happening at the wrong time. What happened to Tracy was normal puberty, but at too young an age. Puberty becomes a medical problem when its timing is wrong. Let's now consider what occurs in normal puberty, with a view to understanding its disorders.

Normal Puberty: What Happens

From a human perspective, the mystery of puberty is that it starts for no apparent reason and transforms our life completely. It is the stuff of myth and poetry. With puberty comes menstruation, also an event with a schedule of its own. And with puberty also comes the possibility of pregnancy.

From a scientific perspective, the mystery is not why puberty starts when it does, but why it does not start sooner. The mechanisms for initiating development and menstruation are present in the infant's brain and pituitary gland, but something keeps them turned off. What that something is has been intensively studied for decades, but we are still far from understanding it.

There are several theories, and each may contain part of the truth. A theory, offered by Professor Rose Frish, promoted the idea that puberty occurs at a specific weight, that somehow the brain senses the body mass or fat mass and lets puberty start when a certain size is reached. This would explain the tendency for petite girls to develop later than tall ones. It would also explain why some women stop getting their periods when they lose too much weight, since they have gone below the body size necessary for the brain to allow puberty. This has biological plausibility. Survival of the human species requires that reproductive capability wait until the body is physically ready. Puberty should not occur until a female is large enough to carry a pregnancy.

This theory has its problems. Not everyone is the same size at puberty. Not all tall or overweight girls develop early; some even develop late. And there is considerable variation in the timing of the development of smaller girls as well. While body fat stores may be involved in regulating the onset of puberty, there must be other mechanisms involved.

If the why of puberty is quite obscure, what happens in puberty is quite familiar. Every woman has experienced it, and so has first-hand knowledge. But this information has its limitations if your daughter's development is not proceeding by a schedule anything like your own. And most adults do not remember the details of their physical development very clearly. The changes occur at a young age and are taken for granted. It may be helpful to review the events of normal puberty so that you can tell when it is normal or abnormal, and so that you can understand the hormonal events underlying the visible changes in your daughter's body.

Two groups of hormones produce two sets of events that make up puberty. The first are the estrogens, mainly estradiol at this age. Estradiol produces the changes in shape that are so obvious in puberty. The estrogens also cause important internal changes in which the uterus becomes larger and its lining becomes capable of either shedding in menstruation or supporting the developing baby in pregnancy.

The other group of hormones are androgens. As we saw in the preceding chapter, these are traditionally called male hormones but really are present in both sexes. They produce the changes of puberty that are common to both boys and girls: pubic hair, underarm hair and odor, oiliness of the skin. Whether they have any other role in female development is unclear. They probably contribute to the increase in bone and muscle mass that occurs in girls at puberty. But androgens mainly come to a teenage girl's attention when they cause such unwanted effects as excessive hair growth or that most characteristic and unwanted condition, acne. These problems are treated in detail in the chapters on androgenic disorders.

Breast Development, Normal and Abnormal

For most girls, the first event of puberty is the appearance of breast buds. For a smaller number, pubic hair appears first. Breast buds are firm tissue just under the nipple. Often they are slightly tender and may be very uncomfortable if accidently bumped. This is probably due to expansion of the tissues in response to estrogen. Fortunately this sensitivity is temporary. In a thin girl breast buds may be visible early, but in heavier girls they may be obscured by fat. Usually a mother will notice the breast buds soon after they appear, but occasionally it is several months before they are obvious. Over a little less than a year, the buds enlarge and the contour of a breast is evident. The nipple and areola also start to grow at this point to more than 1 cm in diameter. Next the nipple grows further so that it stands out from the contour of the breast itself. Finally the breast grows out so that it forms a smooth outline with the nipple.

These stages are illustrated in Figure 5. The great British student of human growth Professor John Tanner first described these stages. Tanner stage I is the situation of a prepubertal child. Stage II is the bud stage. In stage III, the underlying breast tissue is larger than the nipple. Stage IV, the most distinctive in appearance, shows protuberance of the developing nipple and areola. Stage V is the mature breast. Some adult women remain at stage IV, with some nipple prominence. This is just a variation in body shape and has no particular significance.

Another use of Tanner staging is to tell how much more growth in the size of the breast can be expected. American society places value on a woman possessing large breasts, and some girls become anxious that they will not have as much development as they wish. Rarely one or both breasts will not form at all, and it is important to determine if plastic surgery should be considered. For all these situations, assessment of breast development is necessary and can usually be done accurately by a doctor who is experienced in assessing pubertal development.

I think mothers should try to be sympathetic to their daughters' concerns about breast size; they need not be concerned that this is a sign of an intention to begin sexual behavior. Some of the girls I see because of their worries about breast size are quite shy and not at all interested in serious dating. But they want to have physical evidence of womanhood and to feel that they will be attractive when the time comes to date. It is important that girls be reassured that their physical endowment is adequate and will not cause them to be unpopular. Parents should not endorse values that emphasize looks, but they must understand that teenagers live in a social group that does hold these values and be sympathetic to the stress produced by variations in development.

Figure 5.

A Girl with Precocious Puberty

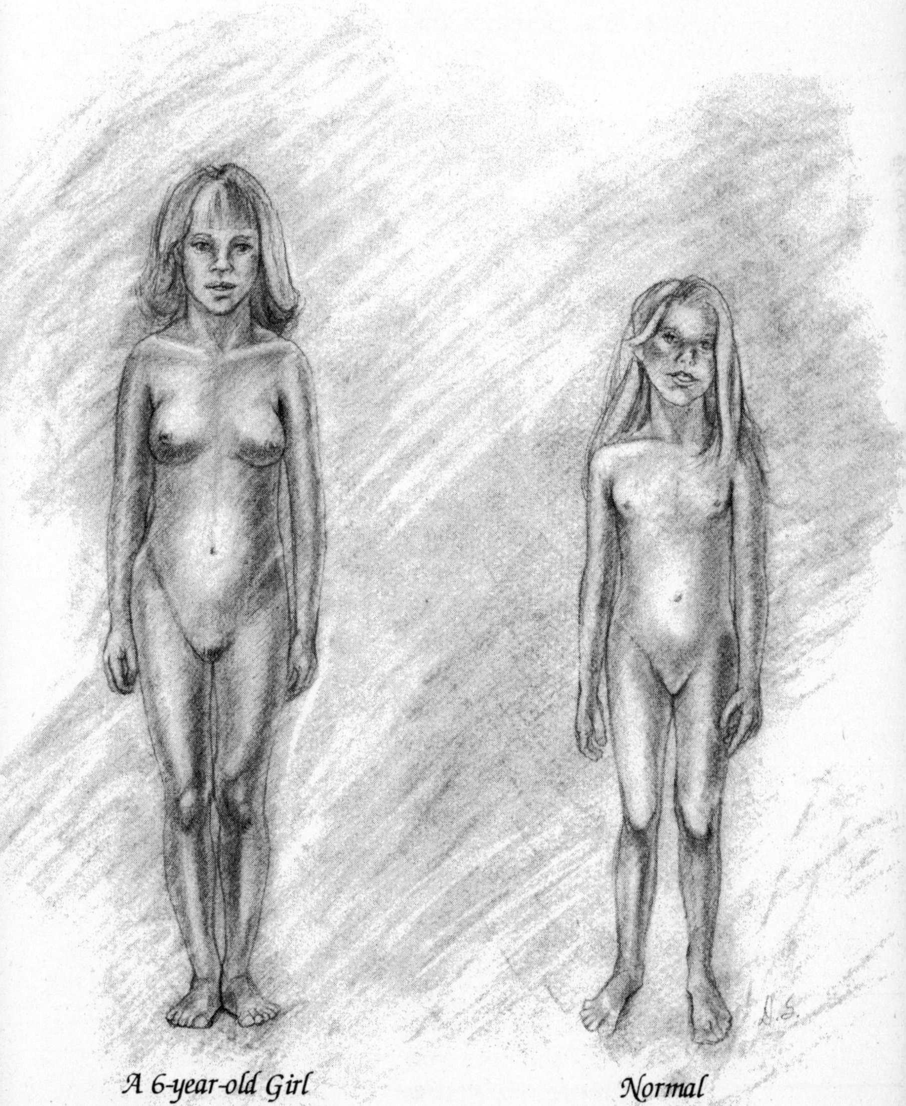

A 6-year-old Girl
with Precocious Puberty

Normal
6-year-old Girl

DISORDERS OF BREAST DEVELOPMENT

Sometimes breasts develop abnormally. Usually the problem is in the breast itself, not in the hormones that stimulate its growth.

While most girls who worry that their breasts are too small either have not yet completed their development or have an exaggerated idea of how big most women's breasts are, some girls do have abnormally small breasts. This is called mammary hypoplasia or aplasia, a condition in which one or both breasts may be very small or not form at all.

Breasts can also be too big. In a condition known as juvenile breast hypertrophy, or mammary hyperplasia, the breasts grow beyond normal size. Sometimes the breast will stop growing when it has reached its mature contour, then start to grow again. This is embarrassing, because teenage girls with large breasts are nearly all teased about it. It can also be uncomfortable, because very large breasts are heavy, and the pull of gravity often makes them sore. Finding clothes that are not too tight on the chest may also be a problem. For a girl with large breasts, mobility is decreased and performance in sports is often adversely affected, especially those that require running. It is no accident that most world-class female athletes are flat-chested.

More common than abnormally small or large breasts is the situation in which there is a discrepancy in size between the two sides. When one breast does not form, the asymmetry is disturbing and may be visible especially with bathing suits or other summer clothing. A common result is avoidance of activities in which the body will be revealed, such as sports. All women have some asymmetry, but it is often so slight as to be unnoticeable. (The same is true of the hands, the feet, and other parts of the body; no one is exactly symmetrical.)

The only treatment for all these variations in breast development is surgery. If breast development is complete and the breasts are still very small, hormonal treatment usually will not help. Hormones only help when there is a deficiency of estrogen, that is, when the problem is delayed puberty. Small breasts are not the result of hormone deficiency, but of something in that person's breast tissue that makes them respond less to the hormone. The same is true of large breasts. The overgrowth is not because levels of estrogen are too high but because of the breast tissue itself. Why some women have breast tissue that grows more than another's during puberty is unknown. Estrogen can make breasts increase in size somewhat, but the effect is slight and the dose of estrogen required is high. In the days when high-dose birth control pills were used, many women noticed a slight but definite increase in breast size, and the breasts went back to their former size when the pill was stopped. But there is a limit to each woman's breast size that cannot be exceeded by increasing the dose of estrogen. In the case of asymmetry, one breast has more growth capacity than the other; the smaller breast has less capacity to respond.

Mothers seldom like the idea of their daughters having breast surgery. Now there is particular concern because of the controversy about the safety of silicone implants. Saline implants seem safer, but because they are used less often there is less information about them. I would offer the following for consideration. First, breast surgery should not be considered until development is complete. This can usually be determined by physical examination by a doctor experienced in problems of breast development. In young girls especially, time may solve the problem as the breasts grow more and as maturity brings self-acceptance. This, however, is not as likely to happen when there is a real abnormality, either marked asymmetry or underdevelopment. In these cases, it may be reasonable to consider surgery, especially for a girl who otherwise will avoid participation in sports or other outdoor activities. Using an insert in one side of the bra may not be satisfying to the affected girl and will not solve the problem when a bathing suit is worn.

In the case of breast overdevelopment, surgery may be the best course. Here, too, it should be delayed if possible until the breasts have definitely stopped growing, because otherwise a second operation may be required. A disadvantage of breast reduction is that sexual sensation in the breasts may be decreased.

Most women I have talked to who have had breast surgery have been happy with the results. This is especially true of those who have had reductions; virtually all feel their comfort and activity have improved. When breasts are extremely small or asymmetrical, it is also reasonable to consider surgery. I feel otherwise in the case of breasts that are normal but not large. If the size of breasts has been greatly increased, the skin often has a stretched look that is not attractive, and the texture of the breast is rather plastic-like. The appeal of breasts is their organic form, and this is altered by implants.

Although attention tends to be focused on the breasts, other parts of the figure, such as the hips and buttocks, can show variation in size and shape. Here again, from an aesthetic perspective, what appeals to one person may not to another. Since estrogen at puberty induces major changes in the shape of the body, it may take several years to see what the end result of these changes will be and for the girl to get used to them. Most of the worries of puberty eventually work themselves out without a need for medical treatments. However, there is a place for intervention when there is a real deviation from normal.

The Other Changes in a Girl's Body at Puberty: Skin and Hair

Pubic hair and underarm hair are emphasized in some cultures but not especially in America. If anything, our culture seems to be averse to these changes. Underarm hair is almost always shaved, and underarm odor, which increases at this time, is not socially acceptable. I am far more likely to see girls who have these events too early or too much than those in whom they are delayed.

Appearance of body hair and body odor with puberty are brought about by androgens. The sources of these hormones in women are the adrenal gland and the ovaries. The adrenal gland is usually the source of androgens in early puberty. Some pre-teenage girls have androgen-mediated changes before their ovaries become active. When the adrenal gland becomes active before the ovary, the result is the appearance of pubic hair, underarm hair and odor, and oiliness of the skin before there is any sign of breast development. This event is called pubarche (designating the appearance of hair over the pubis) or adrenarche (because the adrenal gland has begun to make an adult mixture of hormones).

When pubarche occurs at the expected age, it generally arouses no concern. However, it is not unusual for it to occur at quite a young age. This is called precocious pubarche or precocious adrenarche. Like full precocious puberty, it is a normal event that occurs at an abnormally young age. How young is abnormal? The standard answer is eight years of age, but there are important ethnic differences. Adrenarche is common in black girls at age seven and sometimes younger. It is later in Asian girls. Most often precocious adrenarche shows as early pubic hair, but sometimes the first event is moisture and a hint of adult odor in the underarm area.

With only extremely rare exceptions, precocious adrenarche

is a harmless event. Since the area affected is covered up, other people are not aware and nothing need be done. The girl herself usually does not worry because she is too young to understand the significance of this sort of change. When there is an early appearance of underarm sweating and odor, there may be more concern. This odor is usually quite mild and can be dealt with by daily bathing and use of a deodorant. Some misconceive underarm odor to be the result of lack of cleanliness. This is not strictly true. The action of androgens on the chemistry of sweat results in changes in the normal bacteria that produce the odor. The action of these bacteria is slow and so there is no odor right after washing, but after an hour or two the chemical events produce noticeable odor. Those who do not wash have stronger odor, but even the most thorough washing will not get a girl through the school day without odor. Not all teachers and adults know this, however, and they may wrongly consider a girl with precocious adrenarche to be unclean. For this reason, it is prudent to help a girl with this condition to apply deodorant each morning and to have her bathe frequently. Generally this is all that needs to be done.

However, it is important to be sure that precocious adrenarche is not a sign of something more serious. I have seen many girls with precocious pubarche, but only one or two instances in which the condition was a sign of serious disease, and these girls had other symptoms. Development of more than a few dark hairs on the pubic region is worrisome, especially if there is a very rapid increase.

Fortunately it is quite straightforward to decide if there is a significant hormone problem or not. Physical examination can determine whether it is only a matter of activation of the adrenal gland or whether there is actual puberty, in which the ovary also has started to function. It is important to be sure that the adrenal activation is only to the slight degree expected in early puberty, and not the very high level associated with a hormonal disorder. This is done by measuring the levels of the hormones testosterone and dehydroepiandrosterone sulfate (DHEA-S) in the blood. Because the levels of testosterone in children are hard to measure, it is best if this test be sent to one of the specialized hormone laboratories mentioned in the previous chapter.

At times, there is uncertainty about how rapidly development is progressing. Usually I like to see a girl with early development several times, at about two-month intervals. Development is something that occurs over time, and many situation become clearer over time. Nonetheless I usually do some testing in the beginning so as to not leave grounds for worry.

More About Precocious Puberty

In true precocious puberty, such as Tracey was experiencing, both ovary and adrenal gland become active as a result of stimulation by the pituitary gland. Sometimes the normal brain mechanism that starts puberty is simply switched on at too early an age. Most often, this just happens by itself. Sometimes, however, the brain triggers puberty too early because there is a tumor in or near the hypothalamus, the small area at the base of the brain that controls most hormonal and other basic body functions. These tumors are usually not malignant, but like other brain tumors they can cause damage by pressing on vital structures. Certain of these tumors, called hamartomas, usually do not grow and only need to be watched with periodic MRI scans to be sure they are not expanding. Others, such as germinomas, can often be treated by radiation rather than surgery. Surgery may be needed first, however, to get a sample of tissue in order to identify the tumor and plan treatment. Fortunately these tumors are very rare, but the fact that they can occur is why precocious puberty must be taken seriously

Treatment of brain tumors causing pubertal disorders is complex and beyond the subject of this book. A child with such a problem should be cared for at a center that has a neurosurgeon, neurologist, and pediatric endocrinologist, all experienced with brain tumors in children.

The other serious cause of precocious puberty is tumors of the ovary. Such tumors are exceedingly rare—even rarer than brain tumors—but need to be considered whenever a girl starts to develop breasts before age eight. Sometimes rather than a tumor there is a cyst that produces estrogen for a short time then goes away by itself. Occasionally the ovary will start to function on its own and make estrogen without signaling from the pituitary. This occurs in a condition called McCune-Albright syndrome, or polyostotic fibrous dysplasia. Other glands also may be overactive in this condition, and there are usually birth marks, so-called cafe-au-lait spots, and bone problems associated with it. The spots, the color of coffee with milk, are flat, and may cover several inches of skin. McCune-Albright syndrome is quite rare. Treatment is with drugs, such as tamoxifen, which block the action of estrogen, or testulactone, which stops the body from being able to make estrogen by inhibiting the enzyme aromatase. Currently, these treatments are available as a part of clinical research programs at the National Institutes of Child Health and Human Development in Bethesda, Maryland.

Fewer than 15 percent of girls with precocious puberty have the more serious problems I have just discussed. Most often when precocious puberty occurs it is because the brain simply triggers puberty too soon, and everything else is normal. However, too early development can still have adverse long-term effects on growth, if not treated.

HOW EARLY PUBERTY AFFECTS A GIRL'S GROWTH

Children grow from before birth until the end of puberty when the growth centers of the bones—called epiphyses—close up. After our epiphyses are closed, none of us can grow anymore. It is essential that these growth centers close; otherwise, the bones will be weak in later years. The epiphyses can be seen on ordinary bone X rays as dark lines near the ends of the bones. They are dark on X rays because the epiphyses consist of cartilage where calcium has not yet been deposited.

The sex hormones that produce the physical changes of puberty also act on the epiphyses in the bones to cause the familiar growth spurt of puberty. Testosterone in boys speeds bone growth, but the effect of estrogen in girls is more complex; it has two effects, depending on whether the levels are high or low. Low levels of estrogen stimulate growth, but high levels slow it down. This is why the period of fastest growth occurs fairly early in a girl's puberty, during the year before her periods begin. In boys, the growth spurt comes later but lasts longer.

Anyone who observes children in 7th and 8th grades cannot help but be struck by the wide variation in growth and development at these ages. For a time many girls are taller than the boys, but just as the girls are finishing their growth the boys begin their growth spurt and pass the girls. Considerable anguish befalls many during this process if their growth and development varies from the average. Girls feel awkward to be taller than the boys and the boys likewise are uncomfortable with this situation. While adults know the situation is temporary, time passes more slowly for children, and both boys and girls often feel they will never fit the norms. The ages of twelve through fourteen for girls and thirteen through fifteen for boys are the most difficult in terms of anxiety about one's body and its normality. It is easier to be patient with young people at these ages if one recognizes the tensions they feel.

In considering whether alterations in growth and development may require medical treatment, it is essential to have some idea of what the person's final height will be. The usual rules of thumb, such as the old saw that adult height is twice the height at two years old, are not accurate at all. Fortunately a simple X ray procedure known as bone age makes it possible to determine exactly where a child or adolescent is in her or his physical maturation. Interpreting the bone age makes it possible to predict adult height with reasonable accuracy. Bone age is simply the physical maturity of the body in relation to growth and development, as opposed to chronological age. Thus a girl with precocious puberty will have a bone age older than her chronological age, and a girl who has not started to develop at the normal age will have a bone age younger than her chronological age. The bone age and height prediction are extremely useful in deciding whether growth disorders need treatment, as I shall explain a little later.

How does precocious puberty affect growth? At first, the rise of estrogen in early puberty accelerates growth, just as it does when puberty comes at the normal age. A seven-year-old girl who has the breast development of an eleven-year-old will grow at the rate of an eleven-year-old. This means she will usually be fairly tall for her age. Since a young person's being tall rarely causes adults to worry, this is often unremarked on. However, at the same time this growth spurt is occurring, the growth centers are maturing and preparing to close. In precocious puberty, closure of the epiphyses occurs not at the normal chronological age of about fourteen but at a bone age of fourteen. The girl stops growing when she looks like she is fourteen, rather than later when she actually is fourteen. Parents may not realize that their early-developing daughter, despite being tall now, is at risk of ending up as a very short adult. From time to time, I see a girl who had already finished her growth at a very short adult height as a result of early puberty. This is a very unhappy situation because once the growth centers have closed it is too late to start treatment. Usually the girl's parents had no idea that their daughter's growth was finishing until it actually stopped.

The most lasting effect of precocious puberty is this tendency to stunt height attainment. For this reason, one of the most important parts of medical evaluation of a child with early puberty is prediction of adult height. This can be done with fairly good accuracy with the bone-age X ray. Tables exist for estimating final height based on bone age and present height. This procedure is easy, painless, and essential for your daughter's future well-being if she has precocious puberty.

TREATMENT OF PRECOCIOUS PUBERTY

Truly effective therapy for precocious puberty is a recent advance. Until the mid 1980s, the only treatment available was DepoProvera® (Depo-medroxyprogesterone acetate), a long-acting form of the hormone progesterone that I have discussed in Chapter Two. DepoProvera partially suppresses pituitary release of the hormones FSH and LH, which stimulate the ovary. The problem with DepoProvera is that it only partially turns off puberty at the pituitary level. Although breast development stops and menstruation is prevented, bone maturation continues to advance.

A new class of medications called Gn-RH analogues acts on the pituitary gland to return it to a *completely* prepubertal state. Levels of FSH and LH drop to very low levels so that the ovary is no longer stimulated and stops making the estradiol that causes the pubertal changes in the breasts, bones, and elsewhere. Gn-RH analogues are similar to the brain hormone gonadotropin-releasing hormone, which stimulates the pituitary gland to release FSH and LH. When the pituitary gland is exposed to a constant supply of Gn-RH analogues, however, their effect is the opposite: Release of FSH and LH is inhibited.

Many Gn-RH analogues have been devised, and three are now available in the United States. They are leuprolide (Lupron®, TAP Pharmaceuticals), nafarelin (Synnarel®, Syntex), and histrelin (Suprellin®, Roberts). Leuprolide is available in a depot (long-acting) preparation, which needs to be given only once a month by injection. Nafarelin is a nose spray, but because it needs to be used without fail three times a day, it is not very suitable for small children. At this time, histrelin is only available in a short-acting form that requires daily injections.

With Gn-RH analogue treatment, the return to childhood is almost complete. The breast development does not completely go away, but the tissue softens so much that the breasts become much less noticeable, especially with clothes. When breasts were nearly fully developed before treatment is started, they will not shrink as much but will still be less conspicuous than before.

Pubic hair growth depends on the adrenal gland, not the ovary, and so will not go away with leuprolide and may even increase slightly. Since this is not visible when the child is dressed, it does not present as great a problem.

If precocious puberty has progressed to the point of menses beginning, leuprolide will stop the periods also. This is one of the great advantages of the treatment. Very young girls who have menstrual periods are not usually psychologically harmed by the experience, but it is certainly simpler for all concerned if the periods can be prevented. If a girl with precocious puberty has started menstruation, she will usually have one more period one or two weeks after the first leuprolide injection. Sometimes this also happens to girls who have not yet started their periods but were about to. This is because the uterus has been stimulated by estrogen so that the lining is thick enough to produce a visible amount of menstrual blood when shed. It is not always possible to predict whether bleeding will occur after starting leuprolide, so I always alert the child's mother to this possibility. However, it only happens after the first monthly injection.

Treatment of precocious puberty with Gn-RH analogues has been studied for more than ten years. It appears to be quite safe. Pubertal development resumes once the medication is stopped, so that the girl develops into a normal adult woman. When I was in training in pediatric endocrinology, we were taught that the most important effect of precocious puberty was the shortening of final height, perhaps because this was the part we could not do anything about. The other effects of early development were shrugged off. This lingers on in the belief of some pediatric endocrinologists that treatment with leuprolide is appropriate only when final height will be too short. But, as I thought about this more, it did not make sense. Why subject a very young girl to develop ahead of her peers when there is a safe and effective treatment? It now seems obvious to me that when precocious puberty occurs in very young girls, it should be stopped by treatment. Of course, if puberty is only a little early and not causing any problems, treatment may sometimes not be necessary. But most often it is in the girl's best interest to have puberty occur at the normal age.

LIVING WITH PRECOCIOUS PUBERTY

What happens when it is not possible to stop the progression of puberty in a girl with early development? First of all, it almost always *is* possible to stop it. I would suggest being skeptical of medical advice that treatment is not necessary, at least in any girl younger than seven years old who has started to develop. Whether or not early development is causing immediate problems, there is future height to be considered.

But let's suppose that, for good reason, treatment to stop puberty is not given. While it is usually better to delay puberty to the normal age, the experience of developing early is not as difficult as it might sound. It usually worries the mother far more than the young girl herself. This is because puberty means many more things to an adult than to a child, who has little knowledge about it. When a girl begins to develop early, it does not mean that she will be ready for dating, sexuality, or any of the other new experiences that begin at adolescence. Nor will she think about these matters. A little girl having breasts, hips, and pubic hair—a body that looks nearly adult— does not make her mentally or psychologically an adult. The adults around her such as teachers need to understand this.

The biggest fear that a mother has in this situation is that there will be not only physical but mental precocity as well. Mothers worry that their daughters will start experiencing a sex drive and all the difficulties that go with it. Fortunately this doesn't happen. (At least not with girls; the situation in boys with precocious puberty is different.) In girls with precocious puberty, there does not seem to be an increase in flirtatiousness or any other behavior that seems overtly sexual. It is common for girls with precocious puberty to be irritable and a little more difficult to live with, but sexual issues do not come up. Girls with precocious puberty do have to be protected but this is no different than what prudence requires with other young children—being selective about in whose company they can be left alone. While one might worry that a young girl with a mature body might be more vulnerable to sexual abuse I have never known this to happen to any of my patients with precocious puberty. The crucial factor here is proper supervision. Simply stated, a girl with precocious puberty needs the same adult presence that any other girl of similar age requires.

Whether girls with precocious puberty have *any* of the sexual thoughts that girls have with normal puberty is difficult to know. If they do, such thoughts are not prominent. A young child lacks the words and concepts to understand sexual feelings, let alone explain them to a concerned adult. This is the major reason for the temporary lack of speech of normal adolescence. The mind has so many new kinds of thoughts present that there has not yet been time to learn how to express them. Of course, when puberty is precocious the situation is different. However inarticulate a thirteen-year-old is about her feelings, a three- or a seven-year-old will be even more so. Questioning is more likely to be confusing to the child than informative or helpful. A girl of three or seven with precocious puberty is still a child and will be happiest if talked to and cared for in the manner appropriate for her age. There is no need for premature discussion of sexuality and other adolescent matters.

It is best to explain the situation ahead of time to concerned adults such as teachers, grandparents, and other relatives, who will notice the development. At school, there seem to be fewer problems when the subject is brought up by the mother than if she waits for the teacher to express concern. At times, schools have difficulties dealing with children with special needs. Teachers are usually overworked and undersupported; classes may be too big. One result is that teachers may make up their minds rather quickly about each child and not change these impressions very easily. If your child has special needs, I recommend that you speak to her teacher and the school nurse at the beginning of each school year. They do not need all the details but will be reassured to know that their pupil is under the care of a doctor for her condition; they will be glad to have a basic understanding of what is happening to her. My experience with my patients with precocious puberty is that teachers are nearly always sympathetic and supportive when the child's mother has visited to explain the situation. One reason is that elementary school teachers are usually women and can sympathize with the problems of learning to cope with menstruation, since they have gone through it. I suggest that you explain also that the puberty is physical only and that the girl will not have inappropriately early interest in boys and sex. Rather, the concerns are to minimize embarrassment and to help with menstrual hygiene, which a six- or seven-year-old usually will not be able to handle by herself.

Delayed Puberty

For every girl who startles her mother by developing too soon, there are ten whose mothers worry that they are not developing at all or enough. Delayed puberty is much more common than precocious puberty. While less dramatic than early puberty, late puberty may have even more psychological impact on the girl who is affected by it. (One point of potential confusion should be clarified. Sometimes women joke that they never developed, by which they mean that their breasts are small. Meanwhile they have normal mature breasts that are quite functional. What I am addressing here is the situation where there is truly no development.)

Consider the story of Melissa. She was a few weeks short of seventeen when I first saw her, and she had no physical development at all, or so she and her mother feared. When the other girls started to develop in sixth and seventh grade, nothing happened to Melissa. She and her parents assumed puberty would start sooner or later. Friends and relatives told them stories about "late bloomers" who were behind in their development but began later and ended up more voluptuous than some of their earlier-developing classmates. These relieved the family's worries for a while, but still nothing happened. When her fifteenth birthday passed with no signs of physical maturation, Melissa's mother took her to a pediatrician. He told her that it was normal to not begin menstruation until age sixteen and recommended bringing Melissa back in a year if puberty had not started. It didn't, and the pediatrician suggested seeing an endocrinologist. Actually this was much too long to wait. A girl should be evaluated if she has no breast development by age thirteen or has not started to menstruate by age fifteen.

Although Melissa was embarrassed to see a doctor about such a personal problem, I sensed she wanted to be checked, because the lack of development was a source of worry for her. Each year she had felt more unlike the other girls her age. While precocious puberty is a dramatic event, lack of development is rather a non-event. I quickly reassured mother and daughter that it was a medical problem and did merit full evaluation. I also promised them at once that a way would be found to induce pubertal development, and that Melissa would catch up with her classmates and look like the mature teenager she was.

There was not much more to be learned about Melissa's development. She had always been healthy. She had occasional headaches, but these began in the afternoon and were never associated with nausea. While obviously shy about her condition, Melissa did allow a physical examination after I explained to her what needed to be checked and why. In addition to the usual check of heart, lungs, throat, etc., I palpated her chest to see if she might have some very early breast development. She did not. I also checked the outside of her vagina, where the color of the tissue tells whether estrogen secretion has begun. It had not.

A rectal exam—uncomfortable and somewhat embarrassing for her, but not painful—showed that her uterus and ovaries were present. One concern in lack of puberty is to be sure the normal female internal organs are in fact present. Examination to determine this is extremely important to be able to tell what the effects of the condition will be. An adolescent in such a situation worries whether she will be able to have children, and it is important that she and her mother have specific information about the possibility of pregnancy. While some women choose not to have children, most want to have the option.

Melissa had no breast or pubic hair development, but her uterus was present. It was small, as would be expected because she had not had the estrogen rise of puberty to stimulate its growth. I asked her if people thought she was younger than her age. She said it happened but did not bother her too much. Her family and friends were used to her and liked her, regardless of her problem. But Melissa was concerned about being able to start to date in the future. This first visit occurred in December, and I soon learned in response to my question that the senior prom, now only a few months away, was a worry. Melissa wanted someone to ask her to go, and she did not want to go looking like a little girl.

The average age for an American girl to start breast development is between ten and ten and a half. Most girls—about 95 percent—have started by age twelve and a half or thirteen. If nothing has happened by then, something may be wrong. Usually mothers do not start to worry about a daughter's lack of puberty until she has reached fourteen or fifteen. Melissa's mother did not take her to a specialist until she was seventeen, a situation which is not unusual. This is because most people have an incorrect impression that puberty starts later than it actually does and because there is no exact moment when it becomes abnormal not to have started to develop. Yet if we use menarche as a milestone, no menses by age fourteen and a half or fifteen may be abnormal. The first period is usually two or two and a half years after breast development starts. (It sometimes seems to come more quickly than this because breast development may not be noticed until several months after it has actually begun.)

Puberty is not one event but a sequence and must be evaluated as such. If a girl has not had a period by, say, age sixteen, but breast development started less than three years before and is progressing, everything is likely to be normal. But a younger girl of fifteen who has had not any changes of puberty at all is more likely to have an underlying problem.

Not all girls with pubertal delay have no signs of puberty. Some develop breast buds or a little pubic hair, but then nothing more happens. Or breasts may reach full maturity, but menstruation does not begin when it should. All these situations are of concern and need medical evaluation. All too often, their evaluation is delayed. There are several reasons mothers put off having their daughters evaluated. One is that the situation is an embarrassing one for the girl and sometimes for her mother. Some mothers fear that examination and discussion will be disturbing for their child and postpone it. It can be uncomfortable for the doctor, too. Many physicians feel very awkward about female problems in teenagers. In my experience, this can be as true for women physicians as for male ones. Pediatricians often feel more comfortable with pre-teen patients, internists and gynecologists more comfortable with adult patients.

The outmoded statement still found in textbooks that one need not be concerned about lack of menstruation before age sixteen is sometimes used to put off a necessary but embarrassing examination. If handled sensitively, medical evaluation is far less disturbing to a girl (and her mother) than the uncertainty as to whether she will develop into a woman physically. The time in the doctor's office may involve a few stressful moments, but in the long run the anxiety surrounding that event is less than not knowing what is wrong.

It is very important to choose a physician who will both take the problem seriously and handle it tactfully. I suggest that you find the names of several endocrinologists, either adult or pediatric, but preferably the latter. Then call and ask if the doctor sees many adolescents with this problem and can do the entire workup herself or himself. If the answer is no to either, make inquiries elsewhere. Pediatric endocrinologists have the training to evaluate this situation, but not all are used to doing the examination. In this situation, the individual's personal qualities are as important as board certification, gender, and other more objective attributes. In addition to the above suggestion, I would add that if the physician postpones or avoids a complete evaluation, you should seek an additional opinion.

Genital examination is done differently in an adolescent, especially if she has not been sexually active, than in an adult woman. A Pap smear is not necessary, because the risk of cervical cancer at this age is minute. Unless there have been bleeding problems, insertion of a speculum into the vagina—certainly the most threatening part of a vaginal exam—is not necessary and should not be done. Instead, the outside of the vagina is inspected carefully by the doctor, and the internal female organs are checked by a rectal exam. This is only mildly uncomfortable and embarrassing and also avoids any issues concerning vaginal penetration.

Causes of Delayed Pubertal Development in Girls

Let's return to the story of Melissa's delayed development. Her physical examination showed that while there was indeed no pubertal development, everything else was physically normal. At this first visit, before seeing the lab results I was able to reassure mother and daughter that, whatever the tests showed, Melissa would be able to develop and have her period. This was a great relief to them. The issue of fertility was deferred until I had the results of her hormone tests. Her estradiol was

9 pg/ml, and her FSH and LH were 4.3 mIU/ml and 1.9 mIU/ml respectively, which were in the childhood or early pubertal range. (IU are "international units," which are used for measurement of certain hormones with complex chemical structures.) These results did not tell me if she might eventually go into puberty on her own, but they did tell me something very important. Her ovaries were able to function, otherwise the levels of FSH and LH would be very high because the pituitary would be secreting more in an effort to get the ovary to make enough estrogen. This meant that the problem was either in the pituitary gland or in the hypothalamus, which controls the pituitary.

Melissa did not have enough of the brain hormone Gn-RH, which stimulates the pituitary to make FSH and LH. As a result, she did not have enough FSH and LH in her blood to fully stimulate her ovaries. This condition is called hypogonad-otropic hypogonadism (HH), a cumbersome term that simply means that there is not enough of the gonadotropins FSH and LH to stimulate the gonads (ovaries) to full activity. Before concluding that Melissa had HH, an MRI scan of the hypo-thalamus and pituitary was done to be certain she had no tumor here.

Measurement of FSH and LH is the most important single test in finding the cause of lack of puberty. When the levels are low, as Melissa's were, the cause is in the hypothalamus or pituitary gland. However, if FSH and LH are high, then the problem is in the ovary. The fact that they are too high tells us that the pituitary gland is in overdrive, trying to get the ovary to work.

As I have explained, maturation in a girl is brought about by two groups of hormones: estrogens and androgens. The former stimulates the growth of breasts, hips, and other attri-butes of the feminine shape. The latter causes oiliness of the skin, pubic and other body hair, and underarm sweating and odor. As we have seen, the estrogen-mediated changes are the really important ones, and it is their lack that causes embarrassment and worry. Lack of estrogen is self-evident when a girl has passed the age by which her shape should have changed but no breasts have appeared. If breast development has not started by twelve and a half or no periods have occurred three or more years after breast buds have appeared, then there may be something wrong. I certainly do not mean that all girls who do not develop within these ages have a hormonal disorder; this is definitely not the case. The ages I have given are simply conservative guidelines as to when it is prudent to think of medical evaluation.

HH is a permanent lack of the hormones FSH and LH. However, a much more common situation is simple delayed puberty. In this condition, FSH and LH are low, but eventually the pituitary gland does start to make these hormones, and puberty begins. (Of course, one cannot conclude that there is no underlying problem without the appropriate workup.) Simple delayed puberty has no permanent physical effects but can be psychologically very difficult, because normal teen social activities assume physical maturation. I definitely do not mean sexual activity, but more innocent ones such as swimming or early social contact with boys. Someone who is undeveloped is likely to avoid these activities and may be shunned by agemates. For these reasons, puberty delayed much beyond the normal age needs to be treated.

Sometimes lack of development is attributed to stress or psychological problems. It is true that severe malnutrition or severe stress can retard development. But these causes are extremely rare. Even under the most terrible conditions of war or occupation, girls go on developing. This is not to suggest that psychological factors are not important in the psychological development of adolescent girls. Obviously they are. And stress can have harmful health consequences. But if a girl is not developing physically, it cannot be blamed on stress, on hidden sexual problems, or on bad parenting. Development too early or too late has nothing to do with personal or family problems. Don't blame yourself if your daughter has one of these problems.

Some forms of brain damage—cerebral palsy and related conditions—affect the parts of the brain needed for development. For this reason, it is not unusual for girls with developmental handicaps to start their puberty early or late. These girls often have problems with learning and mobility as well.

There is another problem girls with developmental handicaps can have. This is an inability to handle menstrual hygiene. Problems may result in school or other settings and may make her care more difficult because people outside the family will not tolerate what they see as dirty. In such cases, DepoProvera® can be used to stop menstruation, as well as contraception, if appropriate. Sometimes hysterectomy is suggested in cases like this. Because the girl cannot give consent herself, the ethical issues are complex. For this reason, medication is usually the simplest solution to this problem.

Sometimes lack of puberty is due to a tumor of the hypothalamus or the pituitary gland that damages them to the extent that they cannot secrete their hormones, which are needed for pubertal development. These tumors can be small and at first may produce no other signs than lack of puberty. However, this is very rare; I have seen one or two young people with brain tumors that declared themselves solely by preventing puberty. This possibility makes it necessary to do a full workup on a girl with late puberty. As with other tumors, these usually do less damage if found early. Diagnosis is made by MRI scan.

Girls with HH either do not show signs of puberty at all, or they have some early breast development that does not progress. (When boys have HH, the testicle does not start to enlarge as it should at about thirteen and a half or fourteen, and the other events of male puberty do not occur.) HH is permanent, but it can be treated so as to bring out the normal changes of puberty and, usually, make pregnancy or fatherhood possible. In a form of HH called Kallman syndrome, there is lack of the ability to smell.

Simple delayed puberty is related to a common cause of not getting periods known as hypothalamic amenorrhea. Hormonally it is the same except that it occurs after puberty, so there is lack of menses but not lack of development. I will discuss hypothalamic amenorrhea in the next chapter.

Turner Syndrome and Other Ovarian Problems

I have been discussing situations where puberty does not occur because of a disorder of the brain or pituitary gland. But it can also happen that the ovary fails to form. Without functioning ovaries, a girl will not show any signs of puberty. This is what happens in Turner syndrome, one of the most common of human genetic disorders and one that affects about one in 4,000 girls, not a small number if one considers the number of females in the United States. In Turner syndrome, one of the two X chromosomes is lost during very early development when the embryo consists of only a few cells, and all cells derived from it have only a single X chromosome. For reasons not entirely understood, without the usual second X chromosome, the egg cells in the ovary are rapidly lost so that by early childhood none are left.

The X chromosome does more than determine that a baby will be a girl. Males have an X as well as a Y chromosome and indeed cannot live without the X. Everyone needs at least one X chromosome. Because the X carries the genes for other things, its lack produces other effects besides the too-early loss of eggs from the ovary. The lymphatic circulation does not form fully, resulting in a tendency to puffiness. The hands and feet are usually affected, though the lymphedema, as the swelling is called, is usually not enough to be very noticeable. The skin on the neck is often loose, seemingly due to puffiness of the neck prior to birth. Girls with Turner syndrome may also have abnormalities of their kidneys or heart, although these are usually not serious or are treatable when they are.

The most obvious way in which girls with Turner syndrome differ from other girls is in their growth. In my practice, I see many children because of problems with their growth. Most are boys, because society puts more importance on height for males than for females. So if a girl is brought in because her parents or pediatrician are worried about her growth, she is likely to be extremely short. When girls are very short, it is not unusual for the cause to turn out to be Turner syndrome. Girls with Turner syndrome are normal in size as infants, but their growth does not keep pace with other girls and gradually slows down, making the girl's situation more and more uncomfortable. By thirteen or fourteen, a girl with Turner syndrome is almost always shorter than any of her classmates and has not had pubertal development either. Needless to say, such a situation is very embarrassing for a young teenager.

There are other problems that girls with Turner syndrome face. They are not retarded, but some may need to make an extra effort with math and with certain kinds of spatial problems.

Turner syndrome is diagnosed by growing white blood cells from the patient and examining their chromosomes. If there is only one complete X, the diagnosis of Turner syndrome is made. Most girls with Turner syndrome have only one X chromosome, but some have a piece of the second X or some cells with one X and others with two. This last situation is called mosaicism and tends to produce milder changes. Some girls with Turner mosaicism do go at least partially through puberty. Another helpful test is the FSH level. For reasons described before, it is high in girls with Turner syndrome.

Another name for Turner syndrome is gonadal dysgenesis.

This simply refers to the fact that the gonads—ovaries—did not form normally. There are other, rarer forms of gonadal dysgenesis. In some of these, the gonad has some functioning tissue that can make estrogen. In these cases, the girl may develop partially and even sometimes have periods, although usually these stop at an early age. Some dysgenetic gonads make testosterone as well and may produce some androgenic changes because they have cells with a fragment of a Y chromosome. These conditions are rare and complex and need not concern us here, except to say that when this happens there is a 25 percent chance of a tumor developing in the gonads, so it is necessary to remove them. The chromosome test or other special tests reveal when this surgery is necessary. There is enough variation among individuals with these rare forms of gonadal dysgenesis that if your daughter has one you will need an individualized explanation from her doctor.

There are other conditions besides Turner syndrome that can cause the ovaries not to work. I will discuss these conditions in the next chapter.

When the Internal Female Organs Do Not Develop

Occasionally something goes wrong during a girl's development before birth, and the reproductive organs do not develop. This is called Muellerian agenesis or Rokitansky syndrome. The Muellerian ducts are tubal structures that in female fetuses go on to become the upper genital tract: uterus, Fallopian tubes, and upper two-thirds of the vagina. The lower part of the vagina, including its opening to the outside, develops from other structures. What happens when there is interference with formation of the Muellerian ducts during development depends on how much of the duct was disrupted. In the most complete form, the vagina is very short and there is no upper vagina, uterus, or tubes. In such cases, there can be no menstruation, but external development is normal. In other cases, the uterus is small or abnormally shaped, but there may be some menstruation.

Sometimes the uterus is normal, but there is obstruction to the release of menstrual flow. This can be caused if the hymen has no opening or if there is a vaginal septum, an abnormal membrane sealing off the vagina from the outside. In both cases, it seems as if menstruation has not begun. Actually, however, there will be monthly shedding of the lining of the uterus. There often are menstrual cramps. This condition is easily treated with simple surgery. Unfortunately diagnosis is often delayed because of embarrassment about examining a young girl. Untreated, a blockage in the vagina is not harmless. The menstrual blood, because it is not able to get out normally, flows backward through the uterus and tubes and into the inside of the abdomen. Not only can this cause pain, but the menstrual blood and tissue irritate the internal tissues and can cause the tubes to scar to the extent that they will not be able to function normally. The result may be infertility. In the past, infertility due to tubal factors was particularly difficult to treat. With the development of tubal surgery and in vitro fertilization (IVF), the outlook is better. Nevertheless it is obviously much better to avoid damage to the tubes in the first place.

The Good News About Adolescent Girls' Hormones

For teenagers who have not started to develop, the good news is that it is always possible for the body to mature. Estrogen always works to bring about female development. Although a girl whose body cannot make estrogen will need to take it in pill form, she will develop breasts and hips in the same way any other girl does. Her body does not know that the estrogen came from a pill bottle—nor will anyone else know. Depending on the hormonal medication chosen, blood tests may not be able to tell the difference either. All girls will develop into women, even if they have a hormone deficiency. Most girls so treated will menstruate normally; indeed it is necessary for them to do so to avoid uterine problems.

There are a few situations in which the uterus is lacking and a girl will never get any periods. The best way to help a girl who finds herself in this situation is to explain clearly what has happened, that she will develop a woman's body but that because her uterus did not form she will not have periods. It can be stressed that the other aspects of feminine development will all be normal.

I am not minimizing the problems faced by girls who will be unable to become pregnant. It is an adjustment, and each must come to terms with it in her own way. Parents and doctors can help, but the young person must also think it through for herself. The situation can be presented in the framework of options available to women. While most women elect to bear children, there are many others who do not. Some choose adoption even when they could become pregnant, because they can give a home and a family life to a child who otherwise would not have them.

Infertility treatment has advanced dramatically, and pregnancy is possible for women for whom it was not an option only five years ago. It is possible for a woman with a uterus but not ovaries, as happens in Turner syndrome, to be pregnant. The ovum comes from another woman who donates it, but the sperm comes from the husband. A woman who has ovaries but no uterus can have a surrogate bear a child for her who is genetically her own. This is not an option chosen by many because of the emotional and ethical complexities. But these options do exist. I think it is important for girls lacking a uterus or ovaries to know about these so they know they can have children.

How Estrogen Therapy Can Safely Bring About Development When Puberty Does Not Happen by Itself

In concept, starting development for a girl with delayed puberty is simple. When she takes estrogen, everything will happen that is supposed to happen. Long experience with this kind of treatment in pediatric endocrinology has given a clear idea of the right sequence of doses. Nor is this treatment unnatural. It is normal for a girl's body to have rising levels of estrogen beginning sometime between eight and twelve years of age. Mothers sometimes worry about giving hormones originally intended for adult women to adolescents. However, we now have more than three decades of experience in using female hormones safely in young patients.

The best way for a teenage girl who needs estrogen to start her development is in steps, so that the level rises gradually. The preparation most often used is conjugated estrogen (Premarin®) because with this preparation there is the greatest body of clinical experience in adolescents. (It is also possible to use ethinyl estradiol; studies with this form of estrogen are going on now.) Conjugated estrogen is available in a full range of dosage sizes, so that the exact dose can be selected and there can be flexibility with respect to adjustments. A typical program would be to start at a dose of 0.15 mg, which is one-half of the smallest tablet. After a few months, this is increased to a full tablet, 0.3 mg. At this dose, there are noticeable breast buds, and the breast starts to enlarge after a few more months. After six to twelve months on this dose, the dose is increased further to 0.625 mg. At this dosage level, breast development becomes greater, and the body definitely starts to look more like that of a teenager and less like that of a little girl. On the full dose of 1.25 mg, adult female contours develop. Sometimes the dose is not increased beyond 0.625 mg, but this leaves maturation incomplete for quite a while longer. Girls who have experienced delay in the appearance of pubertal changes are concerned to get to a full adult form and understandably apprehensive about any lingering difference from other girls their age. For this reason, I think it is usually a mistake to keep the dose too low. In days past, doses higher than 1.25 mg were commonly used, but it is now realized that they are rarely necessary.

When puberty is being induced by hormonal treatment, the uterus is ready for its first period when a girl has been on 0.625 mg of Premarin® for a few months. At this point, a progestin is added, which prepares the uterus for shedding. Most often medroxyprogesterone acetate (Provera®), 10 mg daily, is used for the first fourteen days of each calendar month. Bleeding usually begins about two days after the progestin is finished. As with other periods, there may be some moodiness or cramps. A few girls need a slightly higher dose of Premarin to menstruate.

A better understanding of estrogen therapy has made this sort of treatment extremely safe. Earlier problems had to do with using unnecessarily high doses of estrogen and, especially, with not using progestins to induce proper periods. Estrogen replacement is discussed in great detail in Chapter Thirteen.

Normally it takes one to two and a half years to progress from breast buds to the beginning of menses. At this point, the breasts have reached almost but not quite their final adult size. In the schedule of estrogen therapy as outlined above, things are kept close to this timetable. If a girl is older when I see her—say fifteen or sixteen—so that virtually everyone her age is already fully developed, it may be better for her to catch up more quickly. Because of the social emphasis of the senior year of high school, it is especially important to have a girl look her age by this time in her life.

Most of us have not had any say in when we went through puberty; this is the normal state of affairs. I stress this point because I have seen some young people harmed by well-intentioned doctors delaying induction of puberty in the hope that everything will eventually happen on its own. Even worse is to hold off because it is felt the girl is not yet emotionally ready to start puberty. Who of us were? While it may seem that it would be easier to handle puberty when a person is more mature, this means missing the normal milestones of human adolescence and may be harmful in the long run.

Treatment needs to be seriously considered when a girl reaches thirteen without breast development. Many thirteen-year-old girls are not fully developed, but nearly all by this age have at least the beginning of breast development. Not every girl with delayed puberty needs treatment, but all do need evaluation to rule out the kinds of conditions I have outlined earlier in this chapter.

Obviously there are exceptions to any rules one tries to formulate. One such situation occurs when girls or boys are being treated for short stature. In this case, there may be reason to delay inducing puberty to give the bones a longer time in which to grow. Even in this case, puberty should not be put off too long.

Let us see how these principles applied to Melissa. When I proposed to give her hormones to start her development, she nodded agreement that she wanted to do so. Her mother's concerns were more long term. Would the hormones work? Would her development be different on hormones than it would have been if she had developed on her own? Would they cause any side effects or long-term risks? Would she be able to get pregnant and have children? I was able to reassure her on all these issues. As I have stressed above, estrogen therapy produces development identical to that which occurs when estrogen comes from the ovary. It is very safe if done properly. Indeed it is more risky to not take estrogen, because without estrogen calcium is lost from the bones, even in the teens or early twenties. But the psychological risks are even greater. Melissa's mother understood all this.

Melissa's mother also wanted to know what the prospects were for her daughter being able to get pregnant. Here I was able to give very good news. When development does not occur because of a pituitary or hypothalamic problem, special hormonal treatment with gonadotropins (Pergonal® or Metrodin®) is usually necessary to induce ovulation, but the success rate is extremely high.

What were the chances of Melissa being physically more mature by the time of the senior prom? Here I was not able to be as helpful as I would have liked. It was January when all the lab data was back and estrogen was started. The prom was in May. It is possible to give such a high dose of estrogen as to mature the body in that time, but to do so would have been unnatural and, I think, stressful to Melissa. I told Melissa that she would still look younger than her classmates in May, but that she would have definite development by that time. I told her that by the time she started college in the fall, she would look only a little younger than her classmates, and most would probably not notice. Well before the end of her freshman year, she would be fully mature and having periods.

Since Melissa was already seventeen and a high school senior, I felt it would be better for her, as well as safe, if she developed in less than the normal two and a half years. As a result, I started her on 0.3 mg of Premarin® rather than 0.15. I saw her again in April, when I increased her dose to 0.625, a few months sooner than I would have, had she been younger. Melissa was much happier at her visit in April; someone had asked her to the prom. I'm not sure that this had much to do with the fact that she had started to develop. What was most important was the self-confidence she received from knowing that she was not different from all the other girls, that she was starting to develop and would continue to mature. She needed estrogen therapy, but just as much she needed to understand what was happening with her body and to have hope for the future.

Growth Problems in Girls

I have stressed the development of secondary sexual characteristics because they are uniquely related to female hormones. But there is something else just as important in maturation: growth. I mentioned earlier that height is a greater issue for boys than for girls. Eighty percent of patients who receive growth hormone for extremely short stature are males. Many studies show that taller males have advantages in many areas of life: income, achieving promotion, socializing, politics. Height is essential for competitive performance in most sports. Nor is this emphasis on size unique to the United States; there is evidence that being taller has been thought to be better from the beginnings of human civilization. What about girls? Does size matter for them? It definitely does, but the issues are different from the issues for boys. And a girl has to be relatively shorter compared to her peers than a boy to be bothered by it.

Sarah was brought to see me by her mother because she was quite short. This had always been true, even in grade school, but now that she was thirteen, it was starting to bother her more. Sarah's mother thought that she might have some early breast development, but physical examination showed this to be fat, not true breast tissue. Sarah's grades were average, and she was somewhat shy. I suspected this might be due in part to her small size, which makes it harder to feel comfortable asserting oneself in a group. She had friends but was teased about being so short. This teasing bothered her.

When a girl is just petite, but not extremely short, she may like being teased because she interprets it, usually correctly, as an expression of interest from boys. But for very short girls the teasing is too close to home and unwelcome. This was the case for Sarah. Sarah turned out to have Turner syndrome. Her karyotype (chromosome test) showed that she had only one X chromosome, and her FSH was markedly elevated.

Sarah was quite attractive and obviously took care with her clothes. This gave her a doll-like quality that is sometimes appealing to adults but is not good for a teen, who should be treated appropriately for her age. Sarah was not especially interested in sports. Since today there is much more encouragement for girls to be athletic than there was in the past, the limitation shortness imposes on sports performance is now more often of concern to girls. There are certain occupations, such as model, dancer, or flight attendant, that require a certain minimum height. For girls attracted to these careers, short stature can be a great disappointment. For most jobs, it makes no difference. Sarah did not want to be an athlete or a model. She just did not like being extremely short. The average adult height in adults with Turner syndrome is 4' 7", and the tallest girls barely reach 5'. It is easy to understand why Sarah was worried about what the future would bring in the way of growth.

Until recently there was no treatment for the shortness that is part of Turner syndrome. The lack of pubertal development that is part of the disease had been treated all along with estrogen, but the slow growth could not be corrected. However, recent research has shown that growth hormone (GH) can improve growth rate and final height in people with Turner syndrome. Many girls with the condition now reach heights of 5' 1" or taller. With treatment, they may still be petite, but they look normal rather than abnormally short.

Growth hormone can also improve height in girls with other causes of short stature. GH has been controversial, although considering how much it helps children who need it, it is hard to understand why some oppose its use on supposed ethical grounds.

For the first time in human history, it is possible to correct discrepancies in human size. The first question to be considered might be expressed as, "How short is short?" Short is a relative term and may mean different things to different people. To a basketball coach, a height of 6′ may seem short. To a gymnastics coach, a height of 5′ 5″ may seem tall. As a medical problem, shortness can be defined as height below the fifth percentile, which is a standard definition of abnormal in biological measurements. For an adult woman, the fifth percentile is 5′ ½″; for a man, it is 5′ 5½″. Men especially, and some women, who are taller than these heights may consider themselves short and want very much to be taller. However, their height is considered biologically normal.

One of the peculiarities of social attitudes toward short people, especially men, is that while there is considerable discrimination on the basis of height, there is no sympathy for short people. While we educate our children against racism and sexism, there is no effort to make them aware of heightism. Many studies show that taller individuals are more likely to reach high-level positions and that taller men in general have higher salaries. Many people overcome the disadvantage of shortness, but others do not. Shortness is a handicap not because there is anything wrong with being short, but because of the unreasonable discrimination short people face.

Treatment with GH is only to be considered for people who are clearly shorter than the lower normal limit of the fifth percentile. It is not for those whose growth is normal but just want to be taller. For this reason, it is not cosmetic, which refers to changing a normal feature, not to correcting an abnormal one.

With the bone-age X ray it is possible to calculate a height prediction, which will usually tell if a girl or boy will reach a normal adult height or not. If not, then GH can be considered. Although GH is now made with biotechnology, its use in pediatrics is actually not new; it was introduced in 1957. What is new is the unlimited supply of the hormone. Before 1985, GH was made from human pituitary glands obtained at autopsy. All GH now used in the United States is of recombinant DNA origin. There are three preparations: Nutropin and Protropin® (Genentech) and Humatrope® (Eli Lilly Company). All work equally well. In the future other companies may introduce their own brands of GH.

GH is a small protein and would be destroyed in the stomach if taken orally; consequently it must be given by injection six or seven days a week. However, the injections are only under the skin, and the very thin needles on disposable syringes make them virtually painless. If your child goes on GH, you will be taught how to give the shots. Some teens give themselves the injections.

Other than the very rare viral infections that may have come from the old human-tissue preparations, GH has been remarkably free of side effects. Adults with tumors that secrete GH, a condition called acromegaly, often have hypertension, diabetes, and overgrowth of the bones of the face. These effects have been looked for in children receiving GH but have not been found to occur. This is probably because adults with acromegaly have about ten times as much GH as children who receive it by injection. Genentech has a computer database that currently stores information, including side effects, on 13,000 children receiving treatment with GH. It is likely that any serious problems would show up on this, but results so far show GH to be nearly free of problems. Other studies are in progress to improve knowledge of the effects of GH. Because the process of growth occurs over many years, such studies take a long time to be completed.

Several years ago, a Japanese endocrinologist reported that three children treated with GH subsequently developed leukemia. A committee of the Lawson Wilkins Pediatric Endocrine Society and the European Pediatric Endocrine Society was convened to consider the matter. More cases were found; initially there were seventeen, and now there are just over twenty. However, some cases would be expected since leukemia in children, unfortunately, is not rare. Most of the children reported had other known risk factors for leukemia, such as radiotherapy for another form of cancer. At this point, the evidence does not support the idea that GH causes leukemia.

Originally it was thought that only children with a pituitary deficiency of GH would grow better on it. It has now been proved, in many studies from several different countries, that GH does improve growth rates in the majority of children who are abnormally short. Despite this, some pediatric endocrinologists will not treat short children whose GH levels are above a certain arbitrary limit and who do not meet certain other criteria. These criteria were the ones used to ration GH when supplies were scarce and are now outmoded. Unfortunately, doctors are sometimes unwilling to change what they were originally taught. This is an area in which second opinions are often worthwhile. If your child is below the fifth percentile in height and the pediatrician or endocrinologist tells you nothing can be done, it may be advisable to consult someone more experienced with contemporary methods for treatment of growth disorders. GH is certainly not appropriate for all short children, but if height is really troubling your daughter or son, it should be looked into.

Although GH is very expensive, it has generally been covered by health insurance if it is medically necessary, although considerable documentation may need to be provided. This is something pediatric endocrinologists who prescribe GH are used to doing. The anabolic steroid oxandrolone (Anovar®, Gynex) has been used as an alternative to GH for improving growth in children. While safe in the minute doses generally prescribed in this situation, it is not nearly as effective as GH.

Tall Stature in Girls

Because women are "supposed to" be shorter than men, very tall women may find their height embarrassing. Although some very tall girls may appreciate their unusual height, others find it socially awkward. Athletic girls may find height an advantage. Tall males and females are subjected to incessant thoughtless remarks often meant to be humorous. For someone who is a bit shy, the extra attention may be very unwelcome. The problem is at its most difficult in the eighth grade, when children show the widest differences in growth and development.

When a very tall girl is very uncomfortable with her height, it is possible to use hormonal treatment to limit her growth. This usually is not considered unless a girl will grow to be six feet or taller. Estrogen normally causes the growth centers of the bones to close, so that growth ceases. Growth stops much sooner in girls than in boys because high levels of estrogen slow growth as well as mature the bones. Use can be made of this to cause growth to stop ahead of schedule. Somewhat high doses of estrogen are given (usually 7.5 mg per day of conjugated estrogen, together with suitable progesterone replacement, as described in Chapter Thirteen). Treatment is continued until growth is complete as shown by the bone-age X ray. This treatment is safe as long as progesterone is given properly. Menstrual bleeding may be slightly heavy because of the stimulation of the lining of the uterus by the high dose of estrogen. Surprisingly, estrogen side effects like nausea generally do not occur, but it is still best to work up to the full estrogen dose gradually over a few weeks. Problems with thrombophlebitis (blot clots in the leg) have not been reported.

Estrogen treatment of very tall girls has a long history in pediatric endocrinology and is definitely effective. Some pediatric endocrinologists are unwilling to prescribe this kind of treatment because they may not be familiar with estrogen therapy. Adult endocrinologists or gynecologists who use estrogen frequently may not feel comfortable treating adolescents, so it is sometimes hard to find a specialist who will provide this treatment. I suggest that if your daughter is troubled by extreme tallness you call the pediatric endocrinologists near where you live in order to find one who is experienced with its treatment.

Before treatment is planned, your daughter should have a height prediction done on the basis of her bone-age X ray. Often the height prediction shows that a girl who has been worried about her height is nearly finished growing, and she can be reassured that her final height will not be as tall as she had feared. If her adult height will be taller than she is comfortable with, treatment can be considered. Usually heights up to 5′ 10″ or 5′ 11″ are acceptable, but an expected adult height much greater than this may make treatment something to consider. Before starting treatment, it is important to be sure there is no underlying disease causing overgrowth, such as gigantism or Marfan syndrome. A growth specialist can determine this.

It is important to start planning for treatment early, since a girl will continue to grow for a while after treatment is started. Sometime between the ages of eight and ten is about right for the evaluation and planning of future treatment. This does not mean starting hormones at that age, but deciding when will be the best time to begin them. If your daughter is older, it is still possible that something can be done, although the later treatment is started, the less effect it will have on final height.

It is not exclusively girls who sometimes want to limit their height. Some boys are embarrassed by being extremely tall. High doses of testosterone can be used to treat them. There are not many male adolescents for whom being too tall is a worry, and so these treatments are done infrequently.

There is so much variation in human growth and development that all parents at times worry that their child may be abnormal. However, except for delayed puberty, all these problems are uncommon. Most of the time when parents or children worry, nothing more is involved than a variant of normal. If you are concerned, I recommend that you have your child evaluated by a pediatric specialist. If everything is normal, you will be spared further worry. If there is a true disorder, treatment can be started at the optimal time.

Chapter Four
•
Irregular Periods

*T*here is no biological process more mysterious, more steeped in myth, than menstruation. Its coincidence in length with the lunar month, which has never been accounted for in scientific terms, its inevitability, and its uncontrollability give menstruation a seeming power over a woman's destiny. Men are in awe of the process, and at times frightened by its effect on the mood of the women important to them and hence on their own lives.

Anthropology has recently concerned itself with gender issues and there is much fascinating material about differing attitudes and practices regarding menstruation in different cultures. I refer the interested reader to a recent book on the anthropology of menstruation, *Blood Magic*, edited by Thomas Buckley and Alma Gottlieb and published by the University of California Press in 1988.

Tribal and nonmodern societies have very diverse customs regarding menstruation and what women may and may not do during their periods. For example, among the Beng people of West Africa, menstruating women may not go into the forest after they are married, but before menstruation it is permitted. Nor may a menstruating woman tend the fire of another woman. A husband may not eat food prepared by his wife while she is menstruating but may have intercourse with her, though it is not common to do so. The Beng are willing to talk freely about menstruation, though in many other cultures it is a taboo topic. In one Turkish village, girls are never told about the process until their first period, which, for that very reason, is often a traumatic experience. Menstruation is never discussed between men and women, and intercourse is not allowed during menstruation. In many cultures menstruating women are considered polluted, and in Turkey they may not touch the Quran or enter a mosque. They are not allowed to observe the fast of Ramadan, but eat secretly so no one will know that they are menstruating.

A quite different situation exists among the Rungus of Borneo. They have no taboos about menstruation at all. Women do not even use any form of napkin or tampon but sit with their skirts pulled up and their legs covered with a cloth and then, after they get up, use water to clean the bamboo floor. This is as relaxed an attitude as one finds anywhere, although menstruation is not, as other sexual matters are not, discussed between men and women in Rungu society.

Even in our own somewhat permissive culture in which many aspects of sexuality are discussed freely, discussion of periods when men are present is usually avoided. Men usually find the subject more embarrassing than do women. Many Americans abstain from intercourse during menstruation, as often because of the man's preference as well as the woman's. An example of a menstrual taboo, seemingly scientific but actually not, which survives in our society, is the unwillingness of some gynecologists to do a pap smear during a patient's period even though paps done then can be interpreted satisfactorily.

Not all views of menstrual blood are negative. In Tibetan Buddhism, the highest enlightenment is obtained by a complex visualization meditation in which white and red drops representing semen and menstrual blood are united in the central channel of the spiritual body. Here menstrual blood has symbolic significance as the mystical feminine essence. This has been one of the most secret of Tibetan practices; the taboo on discussion of menstruation persists even when it is transformed into a matter of religious significance.

These tribal and ancient ideas about menstruation are fascinating, and help deepen our understanding of this aspect of a woman's life. Yet for contemporary women in the developed countries, the significance of menstruation is rather different. Modern life does not permit allowance for menstruation by decreasing or modifying normal activities. American women still have to work during their periods and to take care of their families. The emphasis has shifted from menstruation being an occasion for a different routine to struggling to keep it from interfering with one's ordinary routine. While the idea of PMS is widely accepted, there is no lessening of expectations of women during this time. Some feminists have criticized the "medicalization" of menstruation. They suggest, for example, that the complaints of women experiencing PMS often represent legitimate concerns that should be addressed rather than abolished with medication. For most women today, however, PMS threatens their well-being and treatment may be the only practical solution.

Menstruation has kept some of its mystery in the unfortunate fact that many women still experience obstacles when trying to fully understand or be treated for an abnormality of their cycle. The purpose of this chapter is to take away as much of the mystery as possible so that you can determine whether your cycle is normal and, if not, what might be wrong and what can be done to correct it.

Most women worry at some time in their life about whether

their cycle is normal. The teen years are a time of concern about sexuality and reproduction, but adolescents have so many things to think about that they usually do not keep their minds on menstruation. However, abnormal periods can be a source of recurrent anxiety to a teenage girl that she may not discuss openly with her mother. Once a woman has had her children, she knows her reproductive system works and usually comes to think about it in a more relaxed way. Of course, for some women there are new concerns that arise after childbearing, relating to menopause, excessive bleeding, mood swings, and other problems.

Women worry about their cycles; most only a little bit, some a lot. Sometimes the worries are needless—what seems abnormal actually isn't. At other times, there may be reason to worry, but it is not clear what to do. Frequently women with irregular periods have consulted a physician who did not seem very concerned, but did not convince them that *they* did not need to be concerned. Some women go for years worrying off and on about a menstrual problem, never sure what it means. Books and articles often fail to be much more helpful. They do not explain specifically what is normal and what is not; nor do they explain what it means if a cycle is abnormal.

I am going to be as clear and specific as possible about what a normal cycle is. I will tell you how to tell if your cycle is normal or not and what sort of menstrual pattern needs medical evaluation. Of course I cannot cover every situation and every possibility. The goal of this book is not to make you your own doctor, but rather enable you to understand as completely as possible what may be wrong, why treatment may be advisable, and what your options are with respect to treatment.

Terms Used to Describe Menstrual Patterns

Before discussing menstrual cycles any further, I need to familiarize you with the medical terms used to describe abnormal patterns. *Amenorrhea* means no menstrual flow; *oligomenorrhea* refers to having flow only occasionally. In practice, these terms are relative. Often amenorrhea is defined as having fewer than four periods per year, while oligomenorrhea is more than four but less than eight. For the sake of simplicity, I have generally used the term amenorrhea to refer to any situation in which a woman usually does not get her period.

Amenorrhea is divided into primary and secondary forms. *Primary amenorrhea* refers to never having had a period at all. This is really a disorder of pubertal development and was discussed in the previous chapter with delayed puberty. *Secondary amenorrhea* means that a woman once had cycles but now does not. The disorders that I will be discussing in the first part of this chapter usually cause secondary amenorrhea, but they can cause the primary form if they begin early in the teens.

Other terms refer to too much bleeding. I'll explain these terms later in this chapter when I discuss problems with excessive bleeding.

Pregnancy and Periods

In explaining different kinds of menstrual problems, I am assuming that you are not pregnant. However, far and away the most common reason for a woman to stop getting her period is that she is pregnant. If this is a possibility, you should have a pregnancy test before thinking that something else might be the cause. Pregnancy complications can cause many different bleeding patterns and may be very dangerous. If you have a sudden change in bleeding pattern, you should call your doctor without delay.

How to Tell If Your Cycle Is Normal

Books on gynecology—both lay and medical ones—tend to be arbitrary in their description of the "normal" menstrual cycle. There is nothing inevitable about such descriptions; they are usually just one person's experience and opinion. Better guidelines can be constructed from an amazing piece of research that has never received the credit or attention it deserves. This is the study of Alan Treloar and his research team members Ruth Boynton, Borchild Behn, and Byron Brown. The study was initiated by a graduate student, Esther Doerr, in 1934, and carried on over a period of thirty years by Alan Treloar, Ph.D., who was chief of the Reproductive Anthropometry Section at the National Institutes of Health. He tabulated data on the menstrual cycles of 27,000 women who attended Northwestern University and who had agreed, beginning in their freshman year, to send in menstrual calendars from then until menopause. This monumental study included more than 250,000 cycles. My discussion of normal cycle patterns is based on their work.

The length of a cycle refers to something other than the length of a period. The *cycle length* is the number of days from the first day of bleeding of one cycle to the first day of bleeding in the next. The average is 28 or 29 days. The *length of a period* is the number of days of bleeding in a single cycle, usually about 5.

Cycles tend to get slightly shorter with age. The median length at age twenty is 28 days, but it shortens to 27 days at age thirty, and then to 26 days at age forty. Cycles typically lengthen again in the one or two years before menopause, increasing to 28 and then 32 days respectively. At all ages, more women have slightly shorter than longer cycles.

The normal range in cycle length is much broader in the years just after menstruation begins and again just before it ends. The range for the two years after the onset of menstruation is 20 to 53 days. By age twenty, the range has narrowed to 22 to 39 days. A decade later, it is 23 to 35 days; three years before menopause, it is 16 to 54 days.

Periods tend to get more regular with age until the approach of menopause. Most women vary within 6 or 7 days, with variations of 3 or 4 days between periods being especially common. Of a group of more than 2,000 women in the study, only one had two years in which all periods were exactly 28 days apart.

There are probably racial and other differences in menstrual patterns. Treloar mentions a study showing that Japanese women seem to have a somewhat longer cycle length and perhaps more variation. The differences are small, however. Among American women, some who are very thin seem to have variation in the length of their cycle, which is often longer than 28 or 29 days. Women who are very overweight also have longer cycles and sometimes are anovulatory, a subject I shall return to later in this chapter. Anovulatory cycles are ones which are abnormal because no egg is released.

This information about cycle length can be formulated into a simple guideline: A normal interval between periods is three and a half weeks to five weeks. However, most women have some cycles that are not within these limits. The question of whether a cycle is abnormal refers to the usual length of your cycle. A longer or shorter one once in a while is common and entirely normal. But if your cycle is consistently shorter than three and a half weeks or longer than five weeks, it should be evaluated. This later standard is a strict one, however. Some women whose cycles are less than three and a half weeks long are still hormonally normal. If you get a period at least eight times a year, that is probably normal even though your cycles may vary in length.

Evaluation for a menstrual problem usually consists of a physical examination, including a pelvic exam and lab tests. I'll explain the reasons for the tests later as I discuss different kinds of menstrual problems. Beyond this, it is a matter of judgment on the part of the physician as to how extensive a workup you need.

Ovulation and the Hormonal Normality of the Menstrual Cycle

I have been defining normal with respect to menstrual cycles on the basis of statistics. When it is approached this way, a woman is normal if she fits into the ranges I have given based on Treloar's huge study. I started with this approach because it is easy to tell what the timing of your cycle is, but more difficult to know what the hormonal changes are. What is most important is whether the hormonal events are normal. If your pattern is not exactly within the ranges I have given you, but your hormones are obeying the normal pattern, then you still have a normal cycle.

A hormonally normal cycle is one in which ovulation occurs and in which the second (luteal) phase is long enough that a pregnancy could have occurred had the egg been fertilized. One woman I know who has five children used to get her period only a few times a year. Obviously she ovulates in those cycles and is hormonally normal. Why then should she bother with these statistical definitions? It is necessary to get some idea of what is normal without the need for tests being done. If your cycle is within the statistical normal, it is very unlikely that you are not ovulating, and so there is no reason to have a special evaluation.

Finding out whether you are ovulating involves some effort. To do so requires either taking basal body temperatures or having repeated blood draws to measure progesterone levels during the second half of your cycle. Basal body temperatures make use of the fact that, at ovulation, body temperature goes up a few tenths of a degree and stays up until progesterone levels fall again, just before menstruation. You take your temperature orally using a special thermometer (ovulation thermometers are available at drugstores) before getting out of bed each morning and plot it on special graph paper. Whether you use temperature or blood, it is best to do a test for at least three cycles to get an idea of the general pattern. Not ovulating during just one cycle does not mean much, since most women do not ovulate every single cycle.

These procedures are not extremely difficult, but they are not extremely convenient either. Few women do them unless they are necessary as part of an infertility workup. However, if your menstrual pattern is outside the usual ranges I have given, there are circumstances in which these tests can be helpful to you.

The number of days of menstrual bleeding shows less variation than the length of the entire cycle. The usual normal is 3 to 7 days. Eight is usually okay, but more than that definitely needs evaluation. Just as an occasional long or short cycle is nothing to be concerned about, the same is true for an occasionally long or short period. How much blood loss is normal? The usual rule is 60 to 80 ml, but obviously the exact amount lost is impossible to measure. (Sixty ml is 4 tablespoons.) I was always taught that use of up to four or five pads or tampons a day is normal, but since women vary in how often they change them, this is subjective also. Yet most women know—and in the case of teenagers, their mothers know—what is the normal amount and what is excessive.

If you do not ovulate, the small blood vessels of your uterus may not be able to clamp down as effectively, and so you may have a longer or heavier period. Not ovulating is a common cause of heavy bleeding. Persistent heavy or prolonged bleeding needs to be checked out. Some women, out of embarrassment or fear that they will be told they need surgery, put off seeing a gynecologist about bleeding problems. This is unwise. Most bleeding can be stopped within a few days by hormonal therapy; D&Cs are rare these days. D&C stands for dilatation and curettage, an operation in which the inner lining of the uterus is scraped away. It was once used frequently for excessive bleeding, before hormonal treatments were available.

What about spotting or breakthrough bleeding? ("Breakthrough bleeding" is enough to require a pad but less than that which occurs with a normal period.) Usually these are due to a slight temporary fall in estrogen levels in the middle of the cycle. If very light extra bleeding occurs in only two or three cycles a year, it probably can be safely ignored. With heavier or more frequent breakthrough bleeding, a checkup is wise. Light bleeding while on birth control pills is common, especially in the first few cycles, and is simply an inconvenience; it is not due to anything wrong with your hormones. Bleeding on the pill is discussed more fully in the chapter on oral contraceptives.

Some Women and Their Cycles

Let me tell you about the menstrual patterns of five women whom I have seen in my practice—without saying yet whether they are normal or not.

Megan, a college student, came to me because her primary doctor had felt her thyroid and thought it was enlarged. As it turned out, her thyroid problem was minor and not affecting her at all. When I took her menstrual history, she told me, "I've always been irregular." She told me her periods generally came during the third week of the month, sometimes on the twenty-second, but other times as late as the twenty-fifth. She had not mentioned her concern to anyone but her roommate, who told her she never kept track of her own periods and had no idea of whether they were regular or not. Megan's periods lasted four or five days and were light, with only mild cramps.

Suzanne, who was twenty-six, came to see me for increased hair growth, which was very mild. She was on birth control pills and told me that her periods were irregular; they were usually very light, and she occasionally missed one altogether. Before she took the pill, she thought they were regular, but she could not remember how often they came.

Esther has three children, including fifteen-year-old Diane, who actually was the patient. Diane had a weight problem and missed her period about twice a year. They weren't too worried about this, but after we discussed it, Esther asked me if she could ask a question about herself. She told me that her periods varied greatly in how often they came. She never knew when they would come, and sometimes they were three or four months apart. This had happened less often since her first child, but it was still unusual for her to have a period two months in a row.

Anne came to see me because, at age twenty-eight, she was overweight and wanted to find out if this was due to a hormonal problem. In the last year and a half, she had gained thirty-eight pounds and was understandably quite concerned about this change in her body. She told me she thought her periods were definitely irregular. She had kept a menstrual calendar but had not thought to bring it: "I forgot. Actually I didn't realize you'd need it." In the past year, her periods seemed to come less often than before, and sometimes they lasted more than a week. She thought this had happened about three times. The closest together her periods had been was three and a half weeks, and the longest interval was nine weeks. Most came at about thirty-five to forty-day intervals.

Megan, Suzanne, Esther, Diane, and Anne were all somewhat concerned about their periods but not enough to mention them as a major issue. In this mild level of concern and in their degree of irregularity, they are like many women, not sure their cycles are normal but, on the other hand, not sure there is anything wrong. They were in a state of uncertainty, although none were extremely worried. Still all were relieved to have their menstrual pattern medically evaluated and would have preferred to have had answers years earlier.

Medicine has been in an era of what might be termed menstrual nihilism. There is a tendency to dismiss any pattern as unimportant unless there is major blood loss or a desire for pregnancy. More than a generation ago, the attitude was the opposite. Women were made to worry unnecessarily about subtle changes in their cycles, and effective treatments did not exist. The current tendency of women to ignore variations in their periods is better than being overly concerned, but what is needed is a balanced attitude. The pendulum has swung too far in the direction of ignoring menstrual problems. Many busy women pay little attention to their cycles. I do not suggest being over-concerned, but I think you are better off if you have a clear idea of what is a normal cycle.

Megan's case is an easy one, both from the doctor's point of view and her own. Megan was twenty, and simply had an exaggerated idea of how regular body rhythms are. Our bodies do not work like computers, and biological rhythms always show a certain amount of variation. Each menstrual cycle is a little longer or a little shorter than the one before it. And the rare woman who really has a completely regular cycle never gets it on the same day each month because most months are longer than the 28 or 29 days of the average menstrual cycle. Megan had not been too worried to begin with, so she said, but I sensed she was pleased when I told her that, if anything, her periods were *more* regular than average.

Suzanne's pattern actually had nothing to do with her own hormones. When a woman is on the pill, the hormones in the pill, not her own ovary and pituitary, control her cycle. This is nothing bad; often it is helpful. Menstrual patterns on oral contraceptives reflect the way a woman's individual uterus responds to the hormones in the pill. It is common with contemporary low-dose pills to have very light periods, sometimes even to the point of their not being noticeable at all. This is fine—-there is no reason a woman has to lose blood each month to be healthy—but it can be unsettling if you didn't know it might happen.

Esther's story of having no difficulty getting pregnant despite an irregular cycle is a common one. Many women are able to become pregnant fairly quickly, even though they do not get their periods every month. Clearly Esther often ovulates or she would not have been pregnant. Most likely she is one of the women with cycles longer than six weeks who is hormonally normal.

What about fifteen-year-old Diane? She missed two periods in the past year. Everyone thinks that teenagers have irregular periods, but this is one of those common beliefs that turns out to be false. It is true that some teenagers miss a period or two in the first year. And it is common for the first periods to be a little longer than four weeks apart. But truly irregular periods in the teens are usually abnormal. If a girl gets only a few periods in her first year after starting menstruation, there is a 50 percent chance that this pattern will continue. Diane did get most of her periods, and I think she will be fine. But I advised her mother that if she began to miss periods more often she should have evaluation for a hormonal disorder. I explained it was unlikely there would be a problem, but if there was, it was best to diagnose and treat it early. A teenager's periods should become more regular over time. If they become less regular, it is much more likely that there is a hormonal problem.

Anne's pattern worried me the most. There had been a definite change: Her periods had become less frequent, and some lasted longer than seven days. Both infrequent periods and long ones can be signs of a failure to ovulate. When some women gain a lot of weight, they stop ovulating. Progesterone measurements can tell if a woman is ovulating, but they have to be timed with the period that *follows* them; this is hard to do if you have no idea when your period will come. I suggested that Anne take MPA (medroxyprogesterone acetate, Provera®) for fourteen days. When she did, she had very heavy bleeding with a lot of cramps. This type of reaction to MPA is what happens when the endometrium is too thick; it confirmed my concern that Anne was not ovulating often enough. I explained why she needed to do something about this, and she agreed to take MPA each month. Anovulation carries an increased risk of a form of uterine cancer and is one of the reasons that irregular cycles need to be evaluated. Endometrial cancer is one of the most preventable of all forms of cancer, but to prevent it you must know if you are at risk. I will explain more about anovulation later in this chapter and in Chapter Thirteen.

What Happens with a Woman's Hormones during a Normal Cycle?

Ovulation is simply the release of the egg cell, or ovum, from the surface of the ovary. After ovulation, whether it has been fertilized or not, the ovum travels down the fallopian tube to the uterus. If it has been fertilized, it will normally implant in the lining of the uterus (the endometrium), there to develop into a fetus. If unfertilized, the ovum is simply lost. The emphasis in this book is not on problems with fertility, not because

Figure 6.

The Internal Changes of the Menstrual Cycle

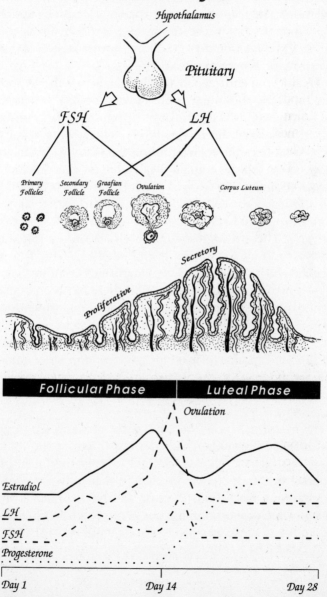

I consider these to be unimportant, but to be able to devote detailed attention to what happens with a woman's hormones when she is not pregnant. Why then bring up the matter of ovulation? The reason is that ovulation is almost as important to a woman who is not trying to get pregnant as to one who is. On ovulation depend certain hormonal events that are necessary for a woman's health.

Ovulation in turn depends on normality of the hypothalamus, pituitary, and ovary, just as puberty does. The hypothalamic hormone Gn-RH stimulates the pituitary gland to secrete follicle-stimulating hormone (FSH), which, as its name suggests, stimulates the follicles inside the ovary to begin to develop. These follicles contain the ova (eggs), one of which will mature enough to be released at ovulation. The action of FSH also stimulates the cells lining the follicle to secrete more and more estrogen into the blood during the first two weeks of the cycle. These rising estrogen levels act on the pituitary to cause a surge of luteinizing hormone (LH). This LH surge triggers ovulation. Another very important event in the ovary follows ovulation and occurs only if there has been ovulation during that cycle. This is called luteinization, which literally means "turning yellow." The follicle, after releasing the egg, becomes a special structure, called the corpus luteum, that has the unique capacity to make progesterone in large amounts. The second half of the menstrual cycle is called the luteal phase because of the presence of this structure that secretes progesterone.

The menstrual cycle, then, has three phases, each of which has different hormonal characteristics. First, in the follicular phase, estrogen levels rise. Second, during the luteal phase, progesterone starts to be secreted so that both estrogen and progesterone reach high levels in the blood. Finally, in any cycle in which conception has not occurred, the corpus luteum becomes less active and progesterone levels drop sharply. Estrogen levels fall also. This is the menstrual phase, when bleeding occurs.

Let's look now at the uterus and how these hormonal events affect it. In the follicular phase, its lining (the endometrium) thickens and new blood vessels form. They are necessary for adequate blood supply for the embryo if a pregnancy occurs. Because of this thickening process, this phase is called the proliferative phase in the uterus and corresponds to the follicular phase of the ovary.

After ovulation, the ovary makes progesterone in the corpus luteum, and this hormone has a profound effect on the endometrium. Microscopic fluid-making structures appear, changing this tissue to what is called the secretory phase. Other changes also make the secretory-phase endometrium able to support a fertilized egg if conception has occurred. There are also important changes in the blood vessels. With progesterone, these develop more muscle cells around them, which enable them to clamp down and limit bleeding if there has been no pregnancy; instead there will be a menstrual period. Progesterone released from the ovary during the days after ovulation prepares the uterus both for pregnancy and for menstruation. This is why ovulation is as necessary for normal periods as it is for pregnancy.

The final phase of the cycle is menstruation. Falling levels of progesterone take away the hormonal support the thickened endometrium needs, and so it breaks down and is shed. Bleeding occurs, as all women know, but it is limited by the chemical and microscopic changes of the secretory phase, which improve hemostasis, the medical term for stopping of bleeding.

Progesterone does not just act on the uterus. It causes fluid retention and, in some women, an increase in appetite. These are part of progesterone's role to prepare a woman's body for pregnancy. But in a cycle that does not result in a pregnancy, as most of the cycles in a woman's life do not, they are not necessary and generally not appreciated by women in whom these effects of progesterone are very strong.

What Can Go Wrong with the Hormonal Events of the Menstrual Cycle?

This background has prepared you to understand what happens in a cycle if the normal hormone changes do not occur. The easiest way to understand menstrual disorders is to consider in turn the two glands involved in the menstrual cycle—the pituitary gland and the ovary—and what can go wrong with each. Note that specific abnormal menstrual patterns that sound similar can be caused by several different hormonal problems. What effect not having periods will have on your health and what treatment is best will depend on the underlying hormone changes.

Hypothalamic Amenorrhea

It is not unusual for the hypothalamus not to release Gn-RH, or at least not enough of it. As a result, the pituitary will not send FSH into the blood, and the ovary will not be stimulated. When this happens, the cycle cannot even get started, and there is no period and no cycle at all. This happens to most women occasionally and to some women fairly often. When it is persistent, it is called hypothalamic amenorrhea. The name reflects the fact that the lack of menses is due to a problem in the hypothalamus. This is a very common form of menstrual disturbance. Factors that seem related to a tendency to hypothalamic amenorrhea are low weight, heavy athletic training, or extreme stress.

The effects of weight, sports, and stress need to be defined more precisely. Many women are slender, athletic, or under stress. Being slender will not usually affect your periods unless you are below ideal body weight. A way you can check if your weight is low enough to affect your cycle is to calculate your body mass index (BMI) as described in Chapter Ten. A BMI of less than 18 or 19 means you may be too thin, and this degree of thinness can cause you not to have your period. This is especially true if you have had anorexia nervosa or bulimia. These kinds of behavior can be very harmful, and you must get professional help if you have them. Calcium loss from the bones is a particular problem with anorexia nervosa and bulimia, because the tendency of the bones to lose calcium when there is estrogen deficiency is made worse by the lack of proper nutrition.

However, some women who have no tendency to anorexia or bulimia are just naturally very thin. Often they are told by well-meaning friends or parents that they should gain weight. If you have a BMI of 19 or greater and get your period every month, you do not have to worry about being too thin. But if you have a low BMI or infrequent periods, then your thinness may be unhealthy. Medical evaluation is a good idea, and you may need to consider estrogen replacement, calcium and multiple vitamin supplements, and efforts to increase your weight. Asian women seem to be able to be thinner than Caucasian women without losing their periods.

Stress can cause periods to become less frequent or stop. This is a form of hypothalamic amenorrhea because stress somehow acts to inhibit release of Gn-RH by the brain. To cause amenorrhea stress has to be truly severe, such as being a prisoner of war or living under other severe threat. Major depression can also cause lack of menstruation, though most women who are depressed still have regular cycles. Events such as starting college or traveling overseas, considered by some contemporary folklore to be likely causes for lack of menstruation, are in actuality not stressful enough to cause amenorrhea. This is important to realize, because if something is wrong with your cycle, you do not want to incorrectly attribute it to stress when that is not the real cause. The same is true of sports participation, which is often wrongly blamed for menstrual problems. For athletics to stop periods, you have to run more than thirty miles a week or train more than two to three hours every day. Track or ballet are more likely to stop periods than is swimming. Weight training is not likely to do so. Normal fitness programs, such as going to an aerobics class several days a week or jogging two or three miles several days a week, will not affect your cycle.

If you are training heavily or are under severe stress and are not getting most of your periods, medical evaluation is still important. You need to be sure that nothing else is wrong, and you probably should have estrogen replacement to protect your bones and maintain the tissue of the vagina in a normal state. Intercourse can cause injury to the vagina if a woman is estrogen-deficient, because it will not have normal thickness and strength or normal lubrication.

I have been describing hypothalamic amenorrhea, in which everything is physically normal but there is a change in function. Most often with hypothalamic amenorrhea this is precisely the situation and nothing more serious is happening. Very uncommonly, however, the hypothalamus and/or pituitary gland are not working because they have been physically damaged. This can happen with severe head injury, with strokes, as a result of excessive blood loss at childbirth, and also with tumors. Tumors in this area can also affect vision; the optic nerves cross just above the pituitary as they travel from the eye to the back of the brain. If the optic nerve is damaged, the field of vision is decreased, but people are not always aware that this has happened. Another sign of tumors is headaches. Of concern are headaches that are present upon awakening in the morning and are associated with nausea or vomiting; these headaches go away completely after someone has been up for a half hour or so. This is not a common pattern. When these occur in children or adolescents, they are often falsely blamed on dislike of school. Morning headaches are not usually psychological and need to be evaluated by a neurologist or, if you are also not getting your periods, by an endocrinologist. Many people wake up with a headache once in a while because they slept with their head at an odd angle or for no particular reason. But if you or your child have frequent headaches in the specific pattern I have described, medical evaluation is needed.

CT (computed axial tomography, also called a CAT scan) and MRI (magnetic resonance imaging) are painless procedures that can determine if there is a tumor in the pituitary-hypothalamic area. Such tumors can be very small, so the films need to be looked at by someone expert in brain radiology. Most tumors in the area of the pituitary can be approached surgically, and some are so slow-growing that surgery is not necessary. If you have such a problem, the best thing you can do is seek out an endocrinologist experienced with pituitary tumors to advise you.

Breast Milk, Prolactin, and Menstruation

A fairly common cause of lack of menstruation is high levels of the pituitary hormone prolactin. The general term for this condition is hyperprolactinemia. As its name suggests, prolactin promotes lactation; it is the hormone that prepares the breast to make milk. Prolactin levels go up somewhat during pregnancy, then rise more dramatically right after childbirth so that the breasts can produce milk. The high estrogen levels of pregnancy cause the lactotroph, the prolactin-making cell of the pituitary, to increase, so much so that the entire pituitary gland expands during pregnancy. Prolactin has another biological function: inhibiting ovulation after childbirth. At that time, a woman's body cannot be ready to have another child right away, and she needs her metabolic resources to be able to breast-feed. Prolactin acts on the hypothalamus and pituitary gland to inhibit release of FSH and LH, and so prevents cycles from starting. It is the mechanism nature has devised for spacing pregnancies. The baby sucking on the breast stimulates continued release of prolactin. This means that menstrual cycles do not usually start again until after the baby is weaned. In biological terms this makes sense. This system is not fail-safe, however. Ovulation is less likely during breast-feeding, but it can occur, and with modern nursing schedules, the baby sometimes does not suck often enough to keep prolactin levels high enough to consistently suppress the menstrual cycle. Nursing works much better as a contraceptive method if the baby is with the mother all day and all night and suckles almost continuously, which is usually impractical in modern America.

What I have described is the normal role of prolactin. In some women, however, prolactin levels are high without relation to pregnancy. In this situation, the effects of prolactin are experienced when they are not expected or appropriate. As you might expect, these effects are the same as occur after childbirth: milk production and lack of menses. Lactation occurring when there has not been a pregnancy is called galactorrhea. This condition is quite common, which should not be surprising; after all, the function of the breast is to make milk. Women who have breast-fed often continue to have very small amounts of milk in their breasts, just a few drops that come out when the nipple is squeezed. Some women who have never had children have small amounts of milk in their breasts, but are not always aware of it. Galactorrhea is important only because it may be a symptom of high prolactin levels. There is no harm in the breast making milk; this is its normal function. However, a few women have enough galactorrhea that it wets their clothes. This is a reason for treatment, although usually galactorrhea needs to be treated only if it is accompanied by lack of menstruation.

If you are having galactorrhea, the first step is to have your prolactin level tested. If your prolactin is normal, then galactorrhea is normal, and nothing need be done about it. (It is best not to keep squeezing your breast to see if milk is still there, as this has the same effect as a baby suckling: It stimulates the breast to make more milk.)

Women sometimes wonder if discharge from the nipple might be a sign of cancer. If it is present in both breasts and is clear or milky, the fluid is not a sign of breast cancer. Clear discharge from one side only is usually nothing to worry about, but having an exam is a good idea. If the discharge is bloody, however, cancer is a possibility, and you need to have a breast exam immediately. Usually breast cancer showing itself in this way has a good prognosis.

What if your prolactin level is high? This indicates a hormonal disorder, especially if you are also not getting your periods. Women who do not get their periods due to high prolactin are estrogen-deficient, and studies have shown that they lose calcium from their bones. Because high prolactin levels stop ovulation, women may first find out they have high prolactin when they are unable to become pregnant; very slight elevations may interfere with ovulation without completely stopping menstruation. Treatment for infertility due to high prolactin is usually successful.

Several situations can cause a woman's prolactin to be elevated. Most women with mild prolactin elevations simply have an increase of lactotroph cells in the pituitary gland. The increase in cells is not enough to be seen on CT or MRI. The next most common cause is a very small tumor called a microadenoma. By definition, microadenomas are entirely within the pituitary gland and measure less than 1 cm in length. They virtually never grow larger and generally cause no problems except the high prolactin. In fact, microadenomas do not behave as tumors and are more accurately thought of simply as a nest of extra cells. Some women (and men) have what look like microadenomas in their pituitary gland, but no change at all in pituitary function. These are called "incidentalomas" in medical slang because they are incidental findings on an imaging study done for another reason. Perhaps one-fourth of women have these tiny, clear areas in their pituitary gland. Most are harmless, but if an MRI or a CT reveals that you have a pituitary abnormality, you should consult an endocrinologist to find out if it is significant or not.

Prolactin elevation can also be caused by macroadenomas. These are larger tumors that have the potential to expand and can harm nearby structures, including the optic nerves. Treatment for macroadenomas is usually effective, but it is best if they are diagnosed before they have expanded. This is one of the reasons it's important to have your prolactin level measured if you are not getting your periods regularly. There may be no other clue to the presence of a micro- or macroadenoma than infrequent or no periods; not all women with high prolactin levels have, or notice that they have, milk in their breasts. When a woman has high prolactin, a CT or, preferably, MRI is needed to distinguish between the different possible causes. Macroadenomas can press on the optic nerves, which cross just above the pituitary gland, and cause loss of vision. If this happens, urgent treatment is required. This sometimes happens in late pregnancy, when very high estrogen levels may cause a macroadenoma to expand. If you have a macroadenoma and become pregnant, you will need to have your vision monitored.

Elevation of prolactin can also occur as an effect of certain medications on a normal pituitary gland. Medications that can increase prolactin levels include such major tranquilizers as chlorpromazine (Thorazine®, SmithKlein Beecham), haloperidol (Haldol®, McNeil), trifluoperazine (Stelazine®, SmithKlein Beecham), prochlorperazine (Compazine®,

SmithKlein Beecham), and others, such as the antidepressants imipramine or amitriptyline, cimetidine (Tagamet®, SmithKlein Beecham), and some (but not most) blood pressure medications. The more common so-called minor tranquilizers sometimes used for ordinary anxiety, such as diazepam (Valium®, Roche), chlordiazepoxide (Librium®, Roche), and alprazolam (Xanax®, Upjohn), do not affect prolactin. If you find out that you have a high prolactin level, the first thing to do is to review with your doctor any medications you are on to see if they might be the cause. Sometimes medication-induced hyperprolactinemia will interfere with the menstrual cycle, but usually it does not. Medications never cause extremely high prolactin elevations, and if your level is over 60 pg/ml, it should not be blamed on medication until a pituitary problem has been ruled out.

TREATMENT FOR INCREASED PROLACTIN

Fortunately hyperprolactinemia (elevated prolactin) is now highly treatable. Special surgical techniques to remove a micro- or macroadenoma were once the only treatment. Now there is a medication called bromocryptine (Parlodel®, Sandoz) that directly inhibits secretion of prolactin by the pituitary gland. If a tumor is the source of the high prolactin, bromocryptine will not only lower the level of prolactin but usually will also shrink the tumor. In fact, it is common for the tumors to go away completely after a few years of bromocryptine. This medical approach has better long-term results than pituitary surgery, and so is almost always preferable. When hyperprolactinemia causes anovulation, bromocryptine usually lowers prolactin to normal and restores ovulation so that pregnancy is possible. If you have high prolactin and want to become pregnant, bromocryptine is the only fertility treatment that will help. It is usually the best treatment for macroadenomas because it will usually stop the tumor from growing any larger and will often shrink it.

There are drawbacks to bromocryptine. Side effects are common, especially in adolescents. The most troublesome is nausea. Some women have dizziness, especially when first starting the drug. Usually these side effects will go away once you are used to the medication, but some women continue to have an uncomfortable degree of nausea. This makes long-term treatment difficult. Yet the estrogen deficiency caused by untreated hyperprolactinemia is itself harmful in the long run. The answer may be to take estrogen replacement instead of long-term bromocryptine. Bromocryptine also may not be the first choice if you are not having periods because of hyperprolactinemia but do not want to become pregnant. If you take bromocryptine, you will start to ovulate again and need contraception. The alternative is to use a low-dose birth control pill, which will provide both estrogen replacement and contraception.

There is an important caution about estrogen in this regard. Estrogen causes the lactotroph cells to increase and the pituitary to enlarge. Estrogen can also stimulate the growth of a macroadenoma since its cells behave like lactotrophs. Only some women with hyperprolactinemia can safely take estrogen—those without a tumor that might expand. Usually estrogen is safe if you have no tumor or only a microadenoma, but this is a decision that must be made with the guidance of an endocrinologist.

In addition to restoring ovulation, bromocryptine also stops galactorrhea. It has also been used to prevent painful breast swelling in women who have just given birth but do not plan to breast-feed. There are rare reports of stroke when it is used in this situation, so safety is a concern.

Doses of bromocryptine range from ½ tablet at bedtime to a tablet three times a day; each tablet is 2.5 mg. Because of side effects, it is best to start with only ½ tablet at bedtime and gradually increase the dosage. The first few doses should be taken when you lie down to go to sleep; you should be very cautious about getting up for the first hour or two after you have swallowed the pill because of the possibility of dizziness and fainting.

I have emphasized the side effects of bromocryptine not to suggest it is a bad drug, but to explain why it is important to work up slowly to the full dose. While nausea is common in adolescents, it is much less common in women in their twenties or older. Most can take the drug without problems, and it has made fertility possible for women who otherwise would never have been able to conceive. And for others it has controlled tumors without the need for major surgery. Bromocryptine has been an important advance in endocrinology.

When the Ovary Stops Functioning Too Early

All women's ovaries eventually stop functioning; this is the familiar event of menopause. While menopause usually happens a little after fifty, it can happen at a much younger age. When the ovary can no longer make its hormones, menstruation stops and other symptoms of lack of estrogen occur. LH and especially FSH levels in the blood are very high at that time because the pituitary gland is trying to stimulate the ovary to function again. When the ovary loses its ability to function before age forty, the situation is referred to as premature menopause or premature ovarian failure (POF). Both terms are unfortunate. While the hormone changes are similar to those of menopause, there is a no premature aging. A twenty-five-year-old with premature menopause is physically like other twenty-five-year-olds, not like a fifty-year-old. She will not age prematurely if she has proper hormone replacement. For that matter, when menopause happens in a fifty-year-old, it does not mean that her body is suddenly much older. The term premature ovarian failure is better, except for its implication that the ovary has done something wrong. I will use the abbreviation POF in referring to this condition, as it is the most emotionally neutral.

POF can have several causes. In menopause, the ovary is depleted of egg cells, and this can happen at an early age. Some women with this form of POF have a mild form of the chromosome disorder that causes Turner syndrome, discussed in the previous chapter.

Some forms of cancer treatment—both chemotherapy and radiation, if it includes the ovaries—cause the ovary to stop functioning. Sometimes the ovaries recover from radiation; however, there is as yet no way to predict whether they will do so. Cancer treatment uses substances that are especially toxic to rapidly growing cells, since cancer cells divide rapidly. The same drugs affect other rapidly growing cells, including the ova. Recently there has been interest in developing treatments for cancers like Hodgkin's disease, which affect women of childbearing age, that will be less likely to destroy the ova. With rare exceptions, drugs other than those used for cancer do not damage the ovary. Hormonal medications do not cause POF.

Autoimmunity is another cause of POF. In autoimmunity, the body's immune system becomes confused and attacks normal tissue as if it were foreign. The ovary may eventually be destroyed, but early on it may only be suppressed by the immune system. Proving that POF is due to autoimmunity can be difficult. A biopsy is definitive but must take tissue from deep in the ovary, and this requires surgery. The specimen must be read by a pathologist experienced with such conditions. Sometimes there are antibodies in the blood that are directed against the ovaries, and these can be measured with blood tests. Only a few laboratories are really able to detect these antibodies, notably that of Professor Noel McClarren at the University of Florida. Autoantibodies against other tissues may also be present, especially those of the thyroid and the parietal cells of the stomach, so testing for these antibodies may help establish that POF is due to autoimmunity.

Pregnancy can sometimes be possible for a woman with autoimmune POF if medications that suppress the immune system are used. The most often used is methylprednisolone (Medrol®), in a high dose of 96 mg per day for ten days or longer. This treatment is not without risks or adverse effects, and only a few infertility specialists and endocrinologists have experience with its use. If you have autoimmune POF and want children, it is the only treatment currently known.

The final cause of POF is a curious condition known as resistant-ovary syndrome, or Savage syndrome. In this condition, the ovary is filled with follicles, the normal structures which surround the egg, but all are in an immature state. They are unable to respond to FSH and LH as they should by enlarging and releasing their eggs. Why this happens is unknown. Sometimes ovulation will start spontaneously, so if you have Savage syndrome there is still a chance you will be able to become pregnant. Among women with this condition, most of the pregnancies have occurred in women taking estrogen and progestin replacement.

POF causes estrogen deficiency, just as menopause does at the more usual age. Estrogen deficiency is even more serious at a young age because bone loss will start very early. If you have POF, or estrogen deficiency from any other cause, it is very important to take hormone replacement. The principles are the same as those for ordinary menopause except estrogen doses should be above the minimum, as younger women's tissues require higher levels. Usually the oral forms work out better for young women because they can be individually adjusted to a greater degree than transdermal estrogen. Medroxyprogesterone acetate, or MPA (Provera®), is used just as it is for menopause. An alternative is to use a birth control pill. This is a good idea if you do not want to become pregnant, since women with POF sometimes ovulate unexpectedly. On the other hand, if you want to be pregnant there is no point in taking the pill because there is sometimes a chance of ovulating while taking estrogen and MPA.

I do want to emphasize that if you have POF it does not mean that you are aging abnormally fast or that you are unhealthy. As long as you take hormone replacement, your body will be like that of other women your age. Occasionally autoimmune POF is accompanied by other autoimmune conditions that can be serious if untreated. If you have POF, consulting an endocrinologist is a good idea.

Lack of Periods and Anovulation

The problems I have described so far occur at the first part of the cycle and keep it from starting at all. Women with these conditions have no or few periods because the endometrium never thickens enough to be shed as menstruation. More common are problems in which the cycle starts out normally. FSH and estrogen rise as they should, but the mid-cycle rise of LH never materializes. Two consequences result. The follicle never releases its egg, and so no pregnancy can occur in this cycle. Without ovulation there also can be no formation of a corpus luteum, and therefore there will be no progesterone in the second phase of the cycle. This situation is anovulation.

Women whose cycles are usually anovulatory menstruate infrequently or not at all, while some have excessive bleeding. This may seem confusing, but need not be if you keep in mind that not all anovulatory situations are alike. If there is little rise in FSH, there will be only relatively low estrogen levels and the endometrium will not get very thick. There may be no bleeding or it will be light. Other women who do not usually ovulate have high levels of estrogen and therefore a thick endometrium and a tendency for heavy bleeding.

One of the effects of progesterone is to prepare the endometrium to be shed normally and to be able to clamp down its blood vessels in order to limit the amount of bleeding that occurs with the period. Without ovulation, there is no progesterone; therefore the small vessels are less able to contract and stop bleeding. For this reason, too much bleeding is a common problem for women who do not ovulate. Over time this tends to get worse because the endometrium becomes overgrown in the absence of progesterone. There may be prolonged spotting or breakthrough bleeding, or regular bleeding may be heavy.

Under the continued stimulation of estrogen without progesterone, the endometrium can become abnormal and eventually cancerous. This happens in stages, over several years. If suspected in time, hyperplasia (overgrowth) of the endometrium can be diagnosed by a biopsy or a D&C, and the uterus can be removed in time to prevent cancer from developing, or from spreading if it has already developed. This is why abnormal bleeding always needs to be taken seriously. Progression from anovulation to cancer of the endometrium can usually be prevented by correcting the situation that causes it: lack of progesterone. Progesterone replacement usually stops the irregular and heavy bleeding and restores regular periods, though it does not restore ovulation. Usually MPA (Provera®) is used for this and is given for at least 12 to 14 days, which is the time the uterus is exposed to progesterone in a normal, ovulatory cycle.

In an ovulatory woman with low estrogen levels, taking a progestin like MPA may not produce any bleeding. When the endometrium is very thick, taking MPA causes a very heavy and often very uncomfortable period. It is like having all the missed periods at once. But the MPA treatment gets rid of the excessively built-up endometrium. Once the endometrium is back to normal, subsequent periods are not terrible, like the first. Using a progestin to shed the overgrown endometrium can prevent further progression toward cancer. This is why all women who are known to not ovulate are put on a progestin or on the pill, which also contains a progestin.

Women who are overweight are more likely to have problems with anovulation, though some women can weigh more than 300 pounds and ovulate normally. Overweight women are also at greater risk for endometrial cancer. I emphasize this because it can be prevented if anovulation is properly treated.

Why is it that some women do not ovulate? This is one of the most challenging research questions in female endocrinology. The problem seems to be in the very delicate interaction between the ovary and the pituitary gland. Instead of LH being released in an abrupt surge in the middle of the cycle, as it is supposed to be, more is released throughout the cycle. Often higher than normal androgens (testosterone and androstenedione) are made in the ovary, and an androgenic disorder results. This is referred to as polycystic ovary syndrome (PCO). This term comes from the presence of many tiny cysts (a cyst is merely a fluid-filled structure, like the bladder), which are follicles that developed but were not able to ovulate normally. Not all women with anovulation have increased levels of androgens and polycystic changes, but many do.

Periods in Perspective

Recently I heard a prominent gynecologist, known for his expertise on menstrual problems, state, "The only predictable thing about the menstrual cycle is its unpredictability." The point he was making is that no cycle is exactly like any other. This is true hormonally; levels of the different hormones vary considerably from cycle to cycle and from day to day during each cycle. Of course, there is some consistency; otherwise ovulation and pregnancy could not occur. Yet biological rhythms do not have the mechanical repetitiveness of mathematical functions. Our bodies are not governed by equations, nor are menstrual cycles. We tend to expect body rhythms to be more regular than they actually are.

Each cycle is a unique event in the life of a woman, not quite like the one before or the one after. There are good cycles and bad cycles. Some bring cramps, mood changes, heavy flow. Others are easy, with little discomfort, no mood swings, and light bleeding. We do not know what subtle hormonal differences make cycles different from each other. An occasional bad cycle or uncomfortable period is nothing to worry about. However, when a problem recurs cycle after cycle, it is usually possible to find out what is happening and to correct it.

Keeping a menstrual calendar is a good idea for any woman with cycle-related problems, because it enables her and her doctor to figure out the pattern and improves the chances of finding the cause of the problem and an effective treatment. Many women feel more comfortable if they are keeping track of their cycles. Other women do not want to bother. If you have no menstrual problem and no concern about pregnancy, it becomes a matter of personal preference whether you record your cycles or not.

THE SIGNIFICANCE OF MISSED PERIODS

I have discussed conditions that cause women not to menstruate, but I have not yet talked about the experience of missing periods. My impression from talking to women is that most (though not all) do not like it if they do not get a period every month. To some physicians, especially males, this seems irrational. To them, the function of the menstrual cycle is to prepare the body for pregnancy. If a woman is not trying to get pregnant, the menstrual cycle has no significance, as long as there is no underlying disease. This rigid attitude is, fortunately, changing. The importance of menstruation for a woman's well-being is becoming more widely appreciated. There is growing recognition of the harmful effects of estrogen deficiency and of the link between lack of ovulation, which is often the cause of lack of periods, and cancer of the endometrium. Not all women who frequently miss periods have either estrogen deficiency or anovulation, although it is important if you frequently miss periods that you find out if you have either of these conditions.

If a woman does not menstruate every month but does not have a hormonal abnormality, do the missed periods have any meaning? Yes. For most women, the regularly recurring cycle is an index of general health. It also reassures about the potential for fertility and the lack of pregnancy. Menstruation means different things to different women and to the same woman at various times of her life.

Some women talk about "backed-up periods." They describe sensations in their body that feel like their period should come, or they wonder if they are having phantom periods that involve hormonal changes but no bleeding. As the term "backed-up period" suggests, some women worry that the blood might be traveling backward into the abdomen rather than being released from the body. They're concerned that this may cause harm because toxic substances are not able to be released from the body.

If you have any of these worries, you can be reassured. Lack of menstruation does not result in accumulation of toxins in your body. Nor is there retention of menstrual fluid, except in very rare conditions in adolescent girls where there is a physical obstruction to the flowing out of menstrual blood. Amenorrhea does not involve the backing up of menstrual fluid. Rather the menstrual fluid is not being formed at all.

A positive aspect of menstruation for a woman can be the sense that it rids her body of something that would otherwise be harmful. It is certainly true that relief from premenstrual symptoms often occurs with the onset of menstruation. So far as is known, however, the cause of this change is not the release of the fluid but rather ~~the fall in progesterone levels that triggers menstruation.~~ Still it is programmed into us to feel better when body fluids are released. The presence of such substances—nasal mucus, thick saliva in the mouth, phlegm in the chest or throat, urine in the bladder, feces in the rectum, or pus in an infected area—is felt as discomfort. With discharge comes a sense of relief. Failure to release these internal substances may result in increased discomfort and fear of harm. This seems to be something very basic in our understanding of our bodies. It is easy to see that, in evolutionary terms, we need instincts to be rid of such discharges. However, lack of a period does not cause harmful substances to remain in your body.

Some women who miss periods feel uncomfortable. They experience this as physical discomfort, heaviness in the pelvis, puffiness, sadder mood, etc. It is easy to say that all this is psychological, and sometimes maybe it is. But there may also be hormonal events like those of normal cycles, but without their rhythmicity. Such hormonal changes are hard to anticipate and therefore may be especially distressing. Cycle-related discomfort is at least predictable. Cramps don't seem quite as bad if one knows they are premenstrual and will get better in two or three days. Similarly, if one knows that an irritable or depressed mood is due to being premenstrual, it at least has an explanation. But for women with irregular periods, the hormonal events are uncoordinated and hence harder to predict or explain. Women with anovulation are more likely to have discomfort or mood changes associated with missed periods than those with hypothalamic amenorrhea or hyperprolactinemia, in which the female hormone levels are fairly constant.

This sort of amenorrhea is easier to tolerate, but it still needs treatment.

The treatment recommended for menstrual disorders when I was a medical student was "reassurance." Sometimes this is, in fact, all that is needed. All too often, however, physician reassurance fails to help for the valid reason that the nature of the problem has not been investigated or explained. Not all menstrual disorders need medical treatment. All do need serious consideration, a diagnosis, and an explanation. And if missed periods are associated with not feeling well, reassurance is not complete treatment.

Most women whose periods are irregular (I mean truly irregular, as explained earlier in this chapter) feel relieved if they can once again have regular periods. To be sure, a few are quite happy not to have to bother with menstruation. Just as there are women who prefer to have periods, there are other women who dislike them. Often I have to convince women that periods are in their best interest, because of the long-term consequences of the hormonal disorders associated with not having them.

TOO MANY OR TOO HEAVY PERIODS

I have given greatest emphasis to conditions that manifest as too few periods. But some women have the opposite: excessive bleeding. This tends to be seen as a more acute problem because it is highly inconvenient and because excessive blood loss is frightening. There are several patterns of excessive bleeding. *Polymenorrhea*, in which periods come too often, can be defined as periods that begin less than three weeks apart. Or periods can last too long (greater than seven or eight days); this is termed *menorrhagia*. With *hypermenorrhea*, periods are of normal length but too heavy. And *metrorrhagia* is bleeding between periods. Lighter bleeding in between periods is usually referred to as spotting or breakthrough bleeding. The latter is enough to require a pad or tampon, whereas spotting is not. Bleeding that is too frequent and too long is called *menometrorrhagia*. I mention these terms because you may encounter them, but they are not terribly useful because they do not contribute to finding the cause of the problem. Sometimes the same condition will cause different bleeding patterns in different women or in the same woman at different times. I have used a simpler classification, which I hope will be clearer.

BLEEDING AND PREGNANCY—A WARNING

Before I go further, I need to repeat my warning that abnormal bleeding can be a sign of a serious complication of pregnancy, such as ectopic pregnancy. If an ectopic pregnancy ruptures, life-threatening internal bleeding can occur. If you are sexually active and have unexpected bleeding that is different from your usual pattern, call your doctor at once. You should do this even if you do not know you are pregnant, because bleeding can be the first sign of pregnancy. Even if you have been using contraception, pregnancy complication is a possibility. Use of IUDs, now rare in the United States, increases the risk that a pregnancy will be ectopic.

PERIODS THAT ARE TOO HEAVY

If your periods do not last more than a week but are very heavy, usually hormones are not involved. Most often this common problem is due to fibroids. Fibroids, more properly but less commonly called myomas (short for leiomyoma), are benign growths of the smooth muscle of the uterus. They can cause it to become enlarged. When they are just under the endometrium (submucosal fibroids), they interfere with the ability of the uterus to squeeze down so as to limit menstrual bleeding. Fibroids grow, like the normal muscle of the uterus, in response to estrogen. Birth control pills, because they contain estrogen, can make myomas grow somewhat larger. Suppression of ovarian estrogen production with a Gn-RH analogue like leuprolide can cause the fibroids to shrink and be easier to remove. If you have fibroids and they are not causing you problems, nothing need be done about them. If they are very large or causing excessive bleeding, or putting pressure on your bladder or creating a heavy feeling low in your abdomen, then surgery may be advisable for you. Sometimes just the fibroids can be removed; in other cases, hysterectomy is necessary. Which is the best procedure for you depends on the size and location of your fibroids and whether you want pregnancy in the future. Fibroids are diagnosed by pelvic exam and ultrasound.

Not all women with very heavy periods have fibroids. To be frank, not much is known about why some women usually have heavy periods and others tend to have light ones. The reason is probably differences in the formation of hormones called prostaglandins within the uterine muscle. These are also involved in causing menstrual cramps. Medications that inhibit prostaglandin formation—the non-steroidal anti-inflammatory drugs (NSAIDs)—usually can decrease the amount of blood lost in a period if everything else is normal. NSAIDs are discussed in Chapter Two.

PERIODS THAT LAST TOO LONG

Most commonly, periods lasting longer than seven or eight days are due to anovulation. Without the effects of progesterone, the uterus cannot stop its bleeding properly, and prolonged menses are a common result. Occasionally fibroids can cause long periods, but usually they make menstruation heavier but not longer. A few women simply have as their natural pattern periods that are longer than what is normal for other women. Before you conclude that menses longer than eight days are normal, it is best to be sure you do not have fibroids and are not anovulatory. I don't want you to think from what I have been saying that there is anything wrong if you have an occasional period that lasts longer than what I have said is normal. If this is only an occasional thing, it is nothing to worry about. It is when long or heavy periods are the rule for you, rather than the exception, that there is reason for concern.

BLEEDING THROUGHOUT THE MONTH

If you bleed all month or most of the month, which may seem like several periods one right after the other, anovulation is the most likely cause. As with any bleeding problem, a pelvic examination is essential to be certain there is no physical abnormality.

Breakthrough bleeding and spotting are milder forms of bleeding and may not be due to an abnormality at all. Mid-cycle spotting is particularly common and may be due to a brief fall in estrogen at the time of ovulation. If it happens only on one or two days and only in mid-cycle, there is no need to be concerned that anything is wrong. This usually happens to women in their teens or early twenties. If you are older than that, spotting is more likely to be due to something else. Breakthrough bleeding is bleeding heavy enough to require a pad or tampon but still much less than a period. Like spotting, it is common in the first few years after menstruation starts, but not later. Breakthrough bleeding can be a normal variant or it can be due to anovulation.

Bleeding can occur after intercourse. Usually this bleeding comes from the cervix, which the penis strikes during thrusting. It is usually simply due to rawness of the tissues on the tip of the cervix, but it can be due to something more serious, such as cervical cancer. If you have post-coital bleeding, you need to have a pelvic exam promptly.

Spotting or breakthrough bleeding is common on the pill, especially in the first few cycles, although it occasionally happens to women who have been on the pill for a year or more. This kind of bleeding is inconvenient but harmless. It is due to the way your uterus reacts to the pill, not to anything wrong with your hormones.

PRE-TEEN AND TEENAGE BLEEDING

Occasionally prepubertal girls bleed from the vagina. Because the blood does not come out immediately, it may be brown in color rather than red. Any brown discharge from a little girl needs to be tested to see if it is blood. The most common cause is a foreign body inside the vagina, most often little bits of toilet paper. However, there can be tumors in this region that show themselves first by bleeding. If your prepubertal daughter has vaginal bleeding, it is essential that she be evaluated by a pediatric endocrinologist or a gynecologist with special training in pediatric gynecology. The sensitive nature of this problem makes it essential that it be handled by a physician who can avoid causing psychological trauma.

When teenage girls have heavy bleeding, it is usually due to anovulation. Most girls outgrow this; in the meantime, it can be controlled by a low-dose oral contraceptive. Occasionally the first period will be extremely heavy; this may be due to a clotting abnormality, and should be evaluated by a gynecologist and hematologist.

TREATMENT OF EXCESSIVE MENSTRUAL BLEEDING

In an earlier era, excessive bleeding often meant that a D&C (dilatation and curettage) was performed. This is a surgical procedure in which the lining of the uterus is scraped off. The opening of the cervix is dilated (stretched open) and the inside of the uterus scraped with an instrument called a curette. D&C takes only a few minutes, but it requires general anesthesia. D&C was used for diagnosis, and the endometrial scrapings were sent for microscopic examination. It also usually stopped the bleeding by removing the thickened endometrium. However, if the bleeding was due to a hormonal problem, it tended to recur. Some unfortunate women were subjected to D&C many times.

Nowadays, D&C is performed infrequently. Endometrial biopsy without anesthesia can be used instead for diagnosis, and hormonal treatment will usually stop the bleeding so that surgery can be avoided. Another procedure, hysteroscopy, involves introduction of a slender optical instrument through the opening of the cervix into the uterus, permitting the gynecologist to see the endometrium and to biopsy abnormal areas. Hysteroscopy needs to be considered when bleeding is very heavy and use of a progestin has not helped. With rare exceptions, you should try hormonal treatment before considering a D&C or hysteroscopy.

A related procedure is endometrial ablation, which is also discussed in Chapter Thirteen. In this procedure, an instrument is put into the uterus with the patient asleep, and the endometrium is removed. Although it usually cures abnormal bleeding, this is a very new procedure, and there is some concern about possible problems. In one such, a condition called adenomyosis, endometrial tissue becomes trapped in the deeper muscle layer of the uterus and can cause enlargement and pain; ablation does not always remove all the endometrium since some of it may be hidden from the surgeon.

Except when due to fibroids, most bleeding problems can be solved without surgery. If bleeding is the result of anovulation, as it usually is, the solution is to replace the missing progesterone. MPA (Provera®) is usually used, though other progestins are occasionally substituted. As discussed in Chapter Thirteen, it is important to take the progestin long enough to completely convert the endometrium from the proliferative to the secretory state. This requires 12 to 14 days of MPA or other progestin. The dose is 10 mg daily, but if bleeding recurs, taking twice this dose for another two weeks may finally bring things under control.

What will happen when you take MPA the first time for a bleeding problem is hard to predict. It depends on the condition of your endometrium, and there is no way to know this. Most commonly, bleeding stops within a day or two after starting the MPA. About two days after MPA is finished, bleeding will start again. This is not more abnormal bleeding but the lining of your uterus being shed, as it needed to be. If the lining had become very thick, the period after MPA may be heavy and uncomfortable. It may also last more than a week. But, most likely, once this is behind you, future periods will be much easier. Sometimes bleeding does not stop on MPA but continues throughout the course of medication and for several days after. Occasionally women bleed during MPA but not after. There is no reason to be alarmed if your bleeding pattern is not exactly as I have described. What is more important is what happens to your period in subsequent months. If you continue to have abnormal bleeding with the use of MPA, you need to be sure you do not have a precancerous or cancerous condition of the endometrium. These conditions can be detected by the procedures just described.

For most women with persistent bleeding problems, the situation tends to recur each month. This is because each cycle is anovulatory. For this reason, it is usually necessary to take MPA each month, as I have described. The most convenient way to remember is to take it the first 14 days of each calendar month. Some women who really hate having periods only use MPA every other month, which is fine if you prefer it. Though taking it less than this often increases the likelihood of problems with excessive thickening of the endometrium. If you can take birth control pills, these may be the simplest way for you to control excessive bleeding.

I wish I could tell you that all problems with excessive bleeding respond to the hormonal treatments I have described. Most do, but some do not. I have stressed that surgery generally should not be the first treatment for bleeding, but if properly used hormonal treatment does not work, surgery may be your best option. Some women put this off as long as possible at the price of being constantly anemic and having to wear a pad every day. This kind of dysfunctional bleeding can be a real handicap. To me, it seems better to have the surgery and put the problem behind you.

I need to repeat my warning that all I have said about bleeding problems assumes you are not pregnant. If you are, bleeding can be an emergency, and the treatment approaches I have discussed may not be proper.

Conclusion:
Hormones and Your Menstrual Cycle

An abnormal cycle can be a sign of something amiss with your female hormones. There is reason for medical concern if there is deficiency of either estrogen or progesterone or both. Estrogen deficiency occurs with hypothalamic amenorrhea, too much prolactin, and premature ovarian failure. The possible harmful effects of estrogen deficiency are like those of menopause: hot flashes, not feeling well, bone loss, and increased risk of heart disease. Treatment is either a birth control pill, as discussed in Chapter Twelve, or estrogen and a progestin, as discussed in Chapter Thirteen.

Progesterone deficiency occurs as a result of anovulation. The risk is of endometrial cancer from overstimulation by estrogen without progesterone. Proper treatment prevents this and consists of progesterone or a related hormonal preparation. Birth control pills have the same beneficial effect, provided there is no reason you should not use them.

If you are not having regular periods, you still have to be careful about contraception. Some women who have very few periods still become pregnant.

While most menstrual disorders do not cause serious health problems, it is still important to have a complete evaluation if you are having fewer than eight periods a year, if you are having excessive bleeding on a regular basis, or if you have any other symptoms that suggest that something is wrong with your cycle. The chances are excellent that your problem can be safely and effectively treated.

Chapter Five

•

Androgenic Disorders: The Most Common Women's Hormone Problem

*Y*ou may be surprised to learn that androgenic disorders are the most common female hormone problem and that their signs are already familiar to you, because androgenic disorders affect women's skin and hair. If you yourself do not have any androgenic problems, you are certain to have a friend who does.

Androgenic disorders affect at least one in ten women, although exact figures are hard to come by because the necessary studies have not been done. One reason most women have not heard the term "androgenic disorder" is because the medical profession has tended to ignore this group of conditions. The result is that most women with an androgenic disorder do not know that this is what they have—though they certainly do know that something is wrong—and are unable to find treatment, even though effective treatment does exist. Androgenic disorders are not only the most common female hormone disorder, they are among the most treatable.

The reason androgenic disorders have been so neglected has to do, unfortunately, with some of the blind spots of the medical profession toward women patients. While the situation has changed greatly for the better—for example, women's concerns about childbirth and breast cancer treatment options are now usually respected—this is least true of the group of conditions grouped under the term "androgenic disorders." Androgenic disorders affect appearance, which our society is hypocritical about, on the one hand judging people by how they look, and on the other criticizing them as vain if they admit they are concerned about it.

I'll begin with the story of Sharon, the twenty-eight-year-old woman whose problem with increased facial hair I told you about in Chapter One. She had first noticed this while in college and the years that followed brought a mild but definite increase in its amount. Sharon would not leave her home or even see anyone until she had removed all visible facial hairs with a razor each morning. Late in the day at work, she could see a grayish coloration on·her chin. Though she invariably made a trip to the ladies' room about two-thirty or three each afternoon to reapply her makeup, she could not escape feeling that the hair growth would be noticed. Sharon told me she would never go out in the evening unless she could go home first to remove her facial hair with a razor. "This is not a normal life for a woman," she told me. "I've come to live with it, but it would seem wonderful just to be able to spend an afternoon at work without having to worry that someone will stand close to me and see the hair growing back. I'd give anything to be rid of this."

A few years before coming to see me, Sharon had tried electrolysis (see page 252). In fact she'd gone for two half-hour sessions a week until she finally gave up. "I spent over three thousand dollars and more than an hour a week for three years before I finally accepted that I was getting nowhere," she said. "When I told the electrologist that I was going to see an endocrinologist, she said it would be a good idea. Why didn't she tell me that before?" Sharon's bad experience with electrolysis is not universal. Electrolysis can be helpful for some women, yet not all electronic hair-removal methods are effective, and it is a procedure requiring considerable skill. For many women with increased facial and body hair, local removal methods like electrolysis or shaving simply are not complete solutions to their problem.

Sharon had seen two doctors about her problem with hair growth, but neither had been helpful to her. The first, a gynecologist she saw shortly after graduation from college, told her she was normal. "I knew it wasn't normal to have so much facial hair," she told me. "I've also always had irregular periods. He just told me not to worry about that until I was married and wanted to have children."

The second doctor was an endocrinologist. "He told me it was too many male hormones. There was a drug he told me about that he said might help with the hair, except that it might cause me to gain weight. That was the end of that for me. But I still think there must be something that can be done about it, even though I haven't found it yet. I'm not willing to give up."

Sharon asked me if I had ever seen anyone else with this problem. She was relieved when I told her I saw between five to ten women every day with increased hair growth and that some had considerably more facial or body hair than she did. Women with increased hair growth usually think they are the only ones who have it. This is because women who have extra hair do everything they can to remove or conceal it.

Ellen's problem with facial hair began, like Sharon's, when she was in college. Unlike Sharon's, however, Ellen's facial hair had increased only slightly. She managed it by bleaching the hairs on her upper lip and plucking the ones on her chin. Ellen had also tried depilatories, but her face would be red and sore afterward. Bleach left her a little irritated also, but not as much as the depilatories. Ellen was not extremely bothered by her facial hair, but she didn't like it. "My mother has it too," she told me. "I'd never thought it was something you go to a doctor about, but one of my friends sees you and so I thought I'd come to see if anything can be done. If not, I'll live with it, but if I didn't have to bleach and pluck, I'd be very happy." Ellen told me that she bleached once a week or less and plucked hairs from her chin two or three times a week.

Keisha is a twenty-three-year-old black woman who works in fashion retailing. She began to notice hair on her upper lip, chin, and sideburns when she was fifteen, and it gradually increased. At first, she didn't mind, and a boyfriend even told her it was sexy. But it has now increased to the point where it is definitely embarrassing to her. At times she has removed it with a razor, but because the hairs often become ingrown as they grow back, she does not do this very often. At times the ingrown hairs would become infected, and Keisha had some darkened areas on her cheeks left over from these infections. Looking me in the eye, she told me she does not set much stock in doctors, but she heard about me from a friend and thought she would check me out.

Our culture just does not admit that females have facial and body hair, even though most women do. Even books on women's health usually do not mention the problem, and those that do dismiss it in a few sentences of generalities. Medicine has shared this denial. Hirsutism (the medical term for increased facial or body hair) is discussed in textbooks, but usually only when it is a symptom of serious underlying hormonal disease, such as an ovarian or adrenal tumor. These are exceedingly rare. Of the more than three thousand women I have seen with androgenic problems, fewer than ten have had such tumors. But women want medicine to offer more than a ruling out of serious disease. They want to understand why they have the increased hair and, most of all, what they can do to decrease it.

I told you a bit about Lenore, a thirty-one-year-old computer programmer who suffered for over fifteen years with acne.

It involved more than pimples; she would develop large red and swollen areas that were painful and healed slowly, sometimes leaving scars.

Several doctors prescribed a series of topicals and oral antibiotics which helped only slightly. She had all but given up hope of ever having clear skin.

Lenore's story is not unique. Seeing a television program I had done about adult acne led her to make an appointment. Before that, she had become quite discouraged. "I'm afraid I may be wasting my time, but I've never been to an endocrinologist, and I thought I'd try one last time. And my mother has been telling me to come. She knows how much it bothers me."

If there is a hierarchy of diseases, acne is the most humble. It is associated with the difficult passage of puberty and, like other problems of the teens, tends to be treated condescendingly by those who outgrew it or never had it. Kids with acne are teased by other teens, and adults often blame them for eating the wrong foods. Adults who have acne feel they have a teenage disease, and this adds to its embarrassment. Yet acne in women is due to a hormonal problem and has nothing to do with diet or lifestyle.

Deanna and her hair loss problem were mentioned in Chapter One. She is twenty-eight and has a lively manner. She likes her job as office manager for a small manufacturing concern. She has a steady boyfriend, but in the last year she has not wanted to go out except to go to work. This is because her hair has gotten thinner, especially in back. She wears her hair in an attractive curly perm; while I could see the thinning that concerned her, it was very mild. When I told her I thought it very unlikely that people were noticing that she had thin hair, she said, "You are probably right, but I can't get the idea out of my head that they are all staring at me. I just don't feel comfortable in public anymore." Deanna was not neurotic, and she did not have a phobia about being out of the house. She'd had none of this reluctance to be seen in public while in high school or in her early twenties. In fact, Deanna was one of my first patients with the problem of alopecia or hair loss. (I will talk about alopecia in Chapter Seven, but I have mentioned Deanna's story here because most female alopecia is due to an androgenic disorder and may accompany acne or hirsutism.)

What Are Androgenic Disorders?

My purpose in this chapter is to give you an understanding of what androgenic disorders are, why they happen, and how they are diagnosed. For many women with an androgenic disorder, the most frustrating thing is to not understand what is happening. The extra facial hair or acne or alopecia is bad enough, but the difficulty in finding out what is wrong with one's hormones makes the condition all the more frustrating. Androgenic disorders primarily affect appearance, but for some women they cause metabolic changes that may increase their risk of serious health problems such as diabetes and heart disease. The effects on both appearance and metabolism can be greatly improved by safe treatments. Androgenic disorders also may affect menstruation and fertility by causing a lack of ovulation. However, the message about androgenic disorders is not a scary one. Rather it is cheerful, because there are good treatments for them. An androgenic disorder is present whenever a woman's body is excessively affected by the family of hormones known as androgens.

Androgens stimulate the pilosebaceous unit, the micro-scopic structure in the skin that includes the hair follicle and the sebaceous glands. The hair follicles grow hair, and the sebaceous glands produce sebum, which is the medical term for the oil of the skin. The biology of the pilosebaceous unit is complex and has not been much studied until recently, because it was not thought to be a site for serious diseases.

Androgens stimulate both sebum production and the activity of the hair follicle. This results in the hair changing from the very fine, almost invisible form known as vellus to the long, thick, opaque body hairs known as terminal. Supposedly all people have the same number of hairs, but most of them are too fine to be visible to the unaided eye. Under the influence of androgenic hormones, however, the vellus hairs become terminal. Appearance of new hair on the body—pubic hair, for example—is not really growth of new hairs but conversion of delicate hairs to ones that are thick and dark enough to be seen and felt. Once activated, the hair follicle goes into a growth phase called anagen. The anagen phase differs in length on different parts of the body. When the anagen phase is long, the hair remains on the body longer, and hair seems thicker and more abundant. After a few months, the hair enters its final phase, called telogen, and no longer grows. After a few weeks, the telogen hair falls out. When so many telogen hairs are lost at the same time as to be noticeable, the shedding is called telogen effluvium.

Let's consider what happens when a woman notices that her facial hair is getting thicker. Actually the hairs do not thicken. Rather new hairs that come in to replace the shed telogen hairs are thicker and darker. So the population of hairs gradually changes. The reverse happens when hirsutism is successfully treated. Under the influence of treatment, the new hairs are lighter and finer. As the old thick hairs reach telogen and fall out, the newer ones that replace them are finer and less visible.

The same structure that makes hair also makes sebum, the oil that appears on our skin in increased amounts, beginning at puberty. Under unfavorable circumstances, sebum cannot escape through blocked pores and a pimple results. The increased sebum production is due solely to the influences of androgens and so *all acne is hormonal*. Failure to realize this results in ineffective treatment for acne. This does not mean that all women with acne have a hormonal disorder. There is a difference between having a disease of one's hormones and having a problem due to hormones. For example, menstrual cramps are caused by hormones, but most young girls who get them do not have a hormonal disease. In most women with acne or increased facial hair growth, the abnormality is not in the blood levels of the hormones or the glands that make them, but in the extreme sensitivity of the pilosebaceous unit to normal levels of androgens. There is something wrong, not with a woman's glands or her hormones, but with the response of her skin to the hormones. This is, in fact, the most common kind of androgenic disorder.

As explained in Chapter Two, androgens are made in the ovaries and adrenals, and both of these become more active at puberty. We know why the ovary makes more hormones at puberty: It is stimulated by the pituitary hormone FSH (follicle-stimulating hormone) and later by luteinizing (LH), also from the pituitary. But we do not know what induces the adrenal gland to change the mixture of hormones it releases into the blood to a higher proportion of androgens. That it does so, however, is well established. At puberty, some girls make higher levels of androgens than others; why this is so is also unknown. It is likely that an undiscovered hormone, probably from the pituitary gland, signals the adrenal gland to increase its production of androgens, but all efforts to find this "adrenarche-stimulating hormone" have so far failed. Yet we can treat excessive androgen production, even though we do not always know what has caused it.

Hormones and Acne

My earlier statement that medicine has neglected the androgenic disorders might seem contradicted by the attention given to acne, which is an androgenic disorder. Acne is the leading reason people see a dermatologist. A variety of prescription drugs have been developed for it, and drugstore shelves are filled with nonprescription acne remedies. Women's magazines frequently carry articles about it. But I still maintain that acne has been neglected as a major cause of mental anguish for women and men who are affected by it. And it has been neglected as an endocrine condition. For acne is not merely a skin disorder. It manifests on the skin but is triggered by hormones. The peculiarities of medical specialization have separated doctors trained to treat skin problems from those trained to treat hormonal problems. Acne is hardly mentioned in textbooks of endocrinology but gets extensive coverage in dermatology books.

Why is this? The simple fact that as medical specialization arose, the endocrine nature of acne was not recognized for the hormonal disorder it is. And dermatologists are used to dealing with skin problems, whereas endocrinologists are not. This situation is unfortunate. Hormones cause acne, and treatment directed at the hormonal cause is most effective. Knowledge from the two specialties needs to be combined for the benefit of acne patients.

Let us look further at how hormones trigger acne. We have already seen that the skin changes of puberty in both boys and girls are due to the actions of androgens. These hormones act on the sebaceous gland to increase its production of sebum. Without androgens, there is only scanty sebum and no acne. The sebum made by the gland has to get out to the skin surface. Often the skin surface protein, called keratin, is too sticky and seals off the opening of the sebaceous gland, so that fluid accumulates in it. This is a whitehead, or closed comedone. If some skin cells are broken down in the process, their pigment gives the comedone a dark appearance and it becomes a black-head or open comedone. Despite what your mother told you—or you tell your daughter—the dark color of a blackhead is not dirt but the normal melanin pigment of the skin. Normally, as the skin renews itself, the top plug falls off and the whitehead or blackhead disappears.

However, in some people a bacterium called *corynebacterium acnes* proliferates in the comedone and converts the sebum to more irritating substances that lead to inflammation. The chemical action also increases the pressure inside the come-done, which may burst inside the skin, leading to the release of the irritating chemicals and a larger and uglier lesion. When these are large, they contain more fluid and are called cysts. (A cyst is simply a fluid-filled structure in the body.)

Acne thus results from a series of steps, beginning with the action of androgens on the sebaceous glands, causing them to produce more oil. Second, the top of the skin is too sticky and the opening of the pore is sealed off. Bacteria grow, causing the oil to become irritating and increasing the pressure inside the pimple. Finally it breaks inside the skin, causing a much larger pimple and considerable inflammation.

The cysts of cystic acne are actually small abscesses or boils. When the cysts finally heal, they leave a small pit or scar. This occurs because new fibrous tissue formed in the healing process pulls the skin, leaving pits, or because the cyst left a small defect in the inner fat layer of the skin. Areas of frequent breakout can become permanently reddened because inflam-mation and the healing process involve more blood flowing through the area. Usually when healing is complete, the exces-sive blood flow stops and the redness goes away. But if there is inflammation nearly all the time, new blood vessels form and may enlarge.

There is a form of acne that affects mainly the nose and the "butterfly" region just next to it; this is called acne rosacea. While the individual lesions are smaller, their location on the tip of the nose makes them especially obvious and hard to conceal. It can resemble another condition that causes too much blood to flow through the skin of the nose: chronic alcohol excess. People with acne rosacea are sometimes thought wrongly to have a drinking problem, which adds to the embarrassment.

Acne usually involves the skin of the face because this is where the pilosebaceous glands are most sensitive to the oil-stimulating effects of the androgenic hormones. But the skin of the upper chest and back also produces sebum, and some people get cystic acne in these regions. Sometimes acne on the shoulders has lesions that are so large that they hurt. Occasionally this happens on the face, too.

The worst form of acne is an uncommon condition called hidradenitis suppurativa. This affects the underarm and groin, and sometimes other skin-fold areas such as the lower breast. In hidradenitis, abscesses or boils form, become swollen and painful, and eventually may drain pus. The infection may be enough to cause fever and often requires treatment with antibiotics and sometimes even surgery. Over time the areas become scarred. Because they do not show, the scars are not the major problem; however, the chronic infection can be debilitating.

While the medical profession has been slow to catch on to the fact that acne is an endocrine disease, women have known for a long time that it is due to their hormones. This is obvious from the fact that acne begins when other hormonal changes do, at puberty, and tends to be at its worst just before periods, when other hormonal events are bothersome.

Everyone's skin becomes oilier with puberty, but not everyone has severe acne. In most people, it gets milder or goes away after the teens, though most women in their twenties and not a few in their thirties get an occasional pimple, especially just before their periods. So hormones and oil production are not the only factors involved in acne. Many women with high androgens make more sebum and therefore are more at risk for acne, but some women have high androgens and very little acne. The other factors are the stickiness of the surface protein of the skin and the particular bacteria growing on the skin. In some, an inherited, more active immune system may produce a greater inflammatory response to acne. Because these factors are so important in the occurrence of acne, they have gotten most of the research attention and the standard treatments are directed at these factors. Antibiotics are commonly used because they inhibit the activity of acne-causing bacteria. And tretinoin (Retin-A®, Ortho) works by making the keratin less sticky. Oral isotretinoin (Accutane®, Roche) works partially in this manner also.

All these approaches have their place, but with the exception of Accutane®, which has problems with side effects, they are not adequate against severe acne. While they are effective to the degree of making the acne milder, they do not result in clear skin. For many women with marked acne, the degree of improvement is not nearly enough. The limitation of all the non-hormonal approaches is that they do not have any effect until the acne process has already started. Obviously it is better to stop acne before it starts, rather than try to ameliorate it later. The hormonal approach stops excess sebum production and so works better than antibiotics or vitamin A derivatives applied to the skin. Without androgen action there is no acne.

Some doctors and others believe that because acne is so common in the teens it is normal. I disagree. Areas of inflammation and infection are not normal. Unfortunately, adolescent concerns may not be taken seriously by adults, which can contribute further to the psychological pain of this difficult time of life. A few whiteheads or blackheads may be normal, in the sense that they do not cause any harm. And a larger lesion once in a while is not a problem. But frequent or plentiful large lesions are not normal and should not be ignored.

Occasionally prepubertal children get acne, usually just on or next to the nose; this is a form of precocious adrenarche (see page 85).

Hormones and Glowing Skin

Even more common than acne is another androgenic effect on skin that does not even have a name. I never was really aware of it until I found it would go away with hormonal treatment. This is a dull appearance to the skin that, like acne, is related to too much sebum production. With this condition, the skin does not necessarily look oily, but simply dull. Normally a woman's skin has a glow that forms part of her attractiveness and appeal. The cosmetic industry is founded on women's wish to enhance this. Hormones are involved in having a glowing complexion, though I have never heard this obvious fact discussed in a medical meeting.

I became aware of the importance of hormones for complexion after seeing that women I was treating for acne or increased facial hair often came back after a few weeks of treatment with truly glowing skin. I suspect that this contributed almost as much to their happiness with the results of treatment as did the clearing of acne or the reduction in facial hair.

When I lecture to doctors, I usually show a few "before" and "after" slides to demonstrate that treatments for androgenic disorders work. One of my favorites is of a woman in her early twenties who came to me for cystic acne, which cleared completely after a few months of spironolactone (see page 227). The audience is always astonished at the change in this young woman's appearance. From looking somewhat mousey, she turns quite radiant. Her acne was not so bad before treatment that she could not conceal it fairly well with makeup. But getting rid of the hormonally induced oiliness literally lit up her face.

A dull complexion may not seem like a medical condition, but for some women it is. In the teens through the thirties and sometimes the forties, dull skin is usually due to too much androgen effect, which leads to too much oil. The skin looks grayish, and the pores enlarge because so much oil passes through them. Young women are often frustrated that a short time after they wash, even if they use a special soap for oily skin, the oil is back again. This is because the androgenic hormones keep the sebaceous glands actively secreting oil. Washing is important but cannot solve the problem because new oil is made after washing. Hot weather makes the sebaceous glands more active and the skin more oily still.

A woman's skin simply looks better if it does not experience too great an androgen effect. Her skin needs estrogens also. When women are estrogen-deficient, as in menopause and sometimes earlier, their skin tends to look thinner or more frail. This is often mistaken to be due to "getting old" but is actually a hormonal deficiency. The need of women's skin for estrogen is discussed in Chapter Thirteen.

Hormones and Facial and Body Hair

The hormonal changes of puberty explain when hair appears but not where it appears. Parts of the body differ greatly in their tendency for hair growth. Everyone, at least initially, has hair on his or her scalp. Almost no one has it on the forehead or on the skin just under the eyes. And, despite the jokes of teenage boys, no one has hair on the palms of the hands. This is because the pilosebaceous units of different skin areas vary in how they respond to hormonal signals. There are also different kinds of hormonal signals. Androgens are the ones that are the best studied and the most important in the hair-growth problems of women, but other biochemical factors that we do not understand also regulate hair growth. This is challenging for researchers but frustrating for the rest of us. Nonetheless enough is known to make sense out of most situations encountered in hair-growth disorders.

Let us examine the distribution of hair on our bodies and its relation to hormones. First of all, a distinction is made between sexual and non-sexual hair. This refers not to any function of the hair or erotic implication, but to whether it grows in response to sex hormones, specifically androgens. Scalp hair and in part the hair on the forearms and legs of girls and boys is non-sexual. So is eyebrow hair. In short, the hair that can normally be seen on the skin of prepubertal children is non-sexual hair. All the rest is sexual hair.

The areas on which androgens can induce hair growth vary greatly in their sensitivity to these hormones. Most sensitive of all is the pubic skin. It is here that hair first appears in the beginning stage of puberty. This skin is most sensitive in the midline and less so to the sides. This is why pubic hair first appears in the middle, along the labia majora in girls and around the base of the penis in boys. As puberty advances, the rising levels of androgens in the blood cause the appearance of dark pubic hairs farther and father to the side. Some women, especially Asians, have a relatively thin band of pubic hair, even when development is complete. Others have pubic hair all the way over to the tops of the thighs. Many women shave off the pubic hair on their thighs because current bathing-suit styles expose this skin, which in current fashion theory is supposed to be hairless but in reality is not. There are also differences in how high on the abdomen pubic hair reaches. Many women have a few hairs between the pubic region and the navel, and some have a band of hair there.

After the pubic region, the next most sensitive area is the underarms, called the axillae in anatomical terminology. This skin shares another response with the pubic skin: It darkens during puberty in response to androgens. This is most notice-able in dark-skinned Caucasians and Asians, but even dark-skinned blacks have darker skin on their pubic and underarm regions. The androgens also make this skin sexually responsive. This is obviously true of the skin of the pubic region but, though unknown to most women and men, the underarm skin is also highly sexually sensitive. Those who like evolutionary

Figure 7.

Places Where Women Can Have Increased Hair Growth

Upper Lip
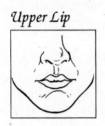

Sideburn Area

Upper Arm
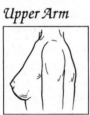

Chin
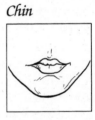

Lower Jaw & Upper Neck
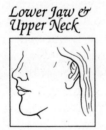

Lower Arm
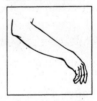

Chest
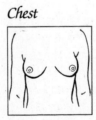

Upper Back

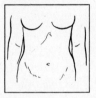

Upper Abdomen

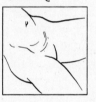

Lower Back

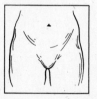

Genital Area & Buttocks

Lower Abdomen

Thigh

Lower Leg

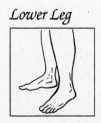

arguments could argue that the hair on these regions serves to draw attention to their erogenous character since arousal is a necessary preliminary to reproduction.

There are differences among women in the amount of axillary hair, but since most American women shave their underarms these are not usually noticed. It is not so in all cultures. Among Asians, who usually have relatively scanty axillary hair, it is usually not removed.

Other areas where hair appears on the body in response to androgens include the small of the back, the lower abdomen, and the chest. A circle of a few hairs around the nipples is normal (though not all women have it), like pubic and axillary hair. The chest, abdomen, and back are most sensitive to androgens in the midline and less so to the sides. In women with increased hair due to the action of androgens, the hair first darkens and thickens in the middle and, if the condition continues to increase, to the sides. Forearm and upper-leg hair is partially sexual (stimulated by androgens) and partially not. Many girls have some hair here before puberty, and it often increases when androgen levels go up.

The amount and distribution of sexual hair is the summation of two factors: the level of androgens secreted into the blood by the ovary and adrenal glands, and the sensitivity of the hair follicle to those hormones. Thus two women with very similar body-hair patterns may not both have elevated androgen levels. One might have high androgen levels and another normal androgen levels, but hair follicles that are very sensitive to these hormones.

Facial hair is also hormonally determined. The most hormonally sensitive skin of the face is the chin, followed closely by the upper lip. The lip differs from most other areas of skin in that it is the outer part—the corners of the mouth—that are more sensitive than the midline. As androgen levels increase or as a woman's skin is exposed to them longer, hair begins to grow closer to the middle of the upper lip. Hair can grow along the lower lip also, but it tends to be lighter and finer than that on the upper lip. Other areas of the face that can have increased hair growth are the sideburns, the cheeks, below the jaw, and the neck. These areas are about equal in sensitivity, but women differ in the tendency of these areas to experience hair growth. Because the chin is so sensitive, probably a majority of women find an occasional thick hair growing from it. The same is true of the corners of the upper lip.

Body Hair in Children

Little girls sometimes have body hair, and their mothers often notice but do not usually worry about it, unless they themselves have had a problem with hirsutism. From time to time, one of my adult patients will ask me about her daughter and tell me, "I just don't want her to go through what I had to go through." This is a natural fear. A mother wonders if her daughter is bothered or embarrassed by facial or body hair and whether it will increase as she matures. The first issue is easier to address. Before puberty, children do not really notice these subtle aspects of their bodies. Young children do not share their mothers' awareness of body hair. If there was anything they minded, it was that it caused a visit to the doctor. Of course, what their mothers worry about is not the present but the future. Here I cannot give blanket reassurance. Visible dark hair on the forearms and lower legs of a little girl may indicate sensitive hair follicles that will become more active once androgen levels rise with puberty. Androgen levels are rather high in the first weeks of infancy and at this time they may prime hair follicles for greater activity after puberty begins.

If you have noticed a tendency to increased hair on your young daughter, however, this is not a reason to be worried. She may never become hirsute. But if the tendency does show itself during her teen development, treatment works better when it is started early. If a teenage girl or her mother starts to notice the appearance of increasing amounts of facial or body hair, it is possible for her to be safely treated to prevent the hair growth from progressing. The medications used are as safe in adolescents as in adults.

The reason few teens are treated for hair-growth problems is the regrettable tendency with all problems in the young to wait and see if they will "grow out of it." The contrary is the case with hirsutism. Hair follicles respond gradually to androgens. Although there is a limit, the longer follicles are exposed to androgens from the blood, the more active they become, the more terminal hair appears, and the thicker and darker the hairs become. For this reason, facial and body hair increases gradually but steadily after puberty. It is several years before the full amount of facial and body hair has appeared.

Some appearance of facial and body hair is a normal part of pubertal development in a girl, but it is one our culture pretends does not occur. We have overcome our modesty about menstruation sufficiently that mothers can prepare their daughters for it. We have not progressed to this point with female hair growth, and I do not see any sign that we will anytime soon. Most doctors do not know about this aspect of female development either, and the advice of pediatricians, however well intentioned, may be inaccurate. Whatever anyone tells you, hair usually increases throughout the teens and into the twenties.

The Natural Course of Hirsutism

The pattern I have described, in which hirsutism begins in the teens, is the most common one, but there are others. Sometimes increased hair appears only at a later age. When this happens, there is also a period of gradual increase over the next several years. Although facial and body hair can start to increase at any age, after her twenties a woman is less likely to start to develop the problem. There are exceptions. Some women start to have it in their sixties.

When hair growth suddenly begins to increase and the increase is so rapid that you can see a change over weeks rather than months or years, the possibility that it is caused by a serious disease must be considered. Doctors worry about this more than patients, though usually unnecessarily; tumors of the ovary or adrenal gland that cause hirsutism are very rare. Of my 3,000 patients with androgenic disorders, fewer than ten turned out to have tumors, and most of these turned out to be benign.

I know that reading books like this often causes people to worry, and I do not want to cause anyone needless distress. If you have had gradually increasing amounts of hair over a few years, you have no reason to worry about a tumor. This does not mean that you should not see a doctor, but that when you do, you are not likely to receive bad news.

Does hirsutism ever get better by itself? I don't think so; if it does happen, it is not very often. However, hirsutism does not always get worse. I have been emphasizing that the amount of hair tends to increase with time, but the main period of increase usually lasts a few years, after which further increase, if any, is slight.

Some women notice that their pubic hair gets more sparse in their forties or later. Why this happens is unclear. It can be an effect of alopecia areata (see page 279). Most often, however, it is probably a result of the normal decrease in androgen levels with age. A few women are embarrassed and fear that husbands or boyfriends will be bothered by the sparseness of their pubic hair. I have never heard of a man minding this and think it is unlikely they will even notice. Treatment with testosterone will probably increase the amount of pubic hair, but it will also increase the hair in other places, so it is usually not worth it.

Many factors account for differences in amount of body hair. There are individual, family, and ethnic differences. The tendency to have a lot of facial or body hair is partly inherited—though this does not mean it is untreatable—but the genetics of body hair in women is not understood very well. Many of my patients tell me that their mothers, sisters, or daughters also tend toward increased facial and body hair, but I also see women with hirsutism whose female relatives are not affected.

There are substantial ethnic differences in body and facial hair. Caucasians have the most, blacks are intermediate, and Asians have least. Among Caucasians, Mediterraneans have more tendency for body hair than other ethnic groups. There are also differences within races in part due to the fact that races have never been genetically completely distinct; intermarriage has occurred since the dawn of mankind.

Non-sexual Hair

So far, I have talked entirely about sexual hair because it is this kind of hair that is hormonally controlled and is most likely to cause problems. But there are conditions in which hair is increased on other areas in which androgens are not involved. Certain areas are almost always free of hair. No matter how high our androgen levels or how sensitive our hair follicles are elsewhere, we do not get hair on our foreheads or on the soft skin just below the eyes. Nor is there hair on the palms and soles or between the fingers or toes, and rarely does it appear on the sides of the trunk.

The main cause for hair growth on places it never normally appears is certain drugs, like the immunosuppressant drug cyclosporin, which for unknown reasons stimulates hair growth in these regions.

Other drugs can cause this increase in non-sexual hair. The most common is the anti-convulsant phenytoin, more widely known by the Parke-Davis brand name of·Dilantin®. An older generic name is diphenylhydantoin. Better medicines with fewer side effects have mostly supplanted this drug. Another causing increases in non-sexual hair is diaxoxide (Proglycem®, Baker Cummins), which is used for low blood sugar problems in children; however these are very rare. Minoxidil is another, and the discovery of this side effect caused the use of the drug to be changed from hypertension to baldness under the brand name Rogaine® (Upjohn).

Appearance and Medicine

So far I have described the hair and skin problems of androgenic disorders with the assumption that they are legitimate medical issues. Some people question whether medicine should concern itself with appearance. It should not be necessary to justify medicine's concern with how people look, but unfortunately it is.

The purpose of hair for humans appears to be decorative and symbolic rather than practical. Hair may keep animals warm, but we do not have enough of it for it to contribute much to protecting us against cold. Skin, of course, is necessary to keep us from drying out and to provide a barrier against infectious organisms. But its decorative function is also evident. Clear skin is prized, even though such changes as scars, blotches, birthmarks, and the like do not make it any less effective in terms of its biological functions. We cannot fully understand skin and hair without consideration of their aesthetic dimension.

Changes in appearance can be harder to live with than internal illnesses which seem more serious. The reason is that changes in skin and hair are there for all to see while most illnesses are concealed inside the body. When they are not, they make the disease much harder to live with.

The few psychological studies that have been done suggest that such problems as acne, though they are rarely seen as serious by those who do not have them, can be very disturbing psychologically to those who do. My own experience listening to the women who come to me as patients confirms this. For the most part, they are well-adjusted people who have managed to prevent the changes in their skin from interfering with their lives, but they nevertheless bear a great burden. In addition to being embarrassed by their visible condition, some also feel guilty that it bothers them so much and worry that they are "vain." When one has worked long enough to have a track record, one is more likely to be judged on actual ability and achievement and less on looks. But appearance is still important if only because of its effect on how one feels about oneself.

I see this again and again in my practice. For example, a woman with increased facial hair may be constantly worried that if colleagues get to close to her at work, they will see the extra hair. Others probably do not notice it, but they might; it is impossible to be sure. When treatment has decreased facial hair to an acceptable amount, an entire area of anxiety vanishes. The woman may look no different to others, but she looks different to herself. In the last analysis, it is how we look to ourselves that is most important.

The Meaning of Hair in Human Life

The peculiar distribution of hair on our bodies is one of our most characteristically human traits. The part of the body that is most fully revealed—the face and head—has the most striking hair pattern of any part.

The presence or absence of hair on the lower face is an area of sexual dimorphism (the scientific term for differences between the sexes). Women do not have hair there and men do, or so we assume. Our culture tends to make these sexual differences more absolute than they really are. For example, we all know women have breasts and men do not. But many men have a small nubbin of breast tissue under the nipple and often a mound of fat.

Just as breasts are not quite so exclusively female as they are usually thought to be, so facial and body hair are not so exclusively male. Daily shaving is thought to be a ritual for all males, yet many Asian and black males do not shave every day. And some women remove facial hair with a razor every day. Shaving seems specifically masculine only in the context of a culture that insists on seeing women and men as absolutely different physically. Yet we are all human, and our bodies are more similar than different. We all have secret traits that we imagine belong to the other gender, and we tend to bear these in silence. When they cannot be concealed, they are far more bothersome.

How Much Hair Is Normal for a Woman?

Many women worry about whether the amount of hair they have is normal or not. There is no precise answer to this question, because there is no precise dividing line between normal and abnormal. Whether the quantity of hair a woman has is significant depends less on the exact amount than on its significance for her well-being. Most important is whether the increased hair represents a sign of serious disease that needs to be diagnosed and treated because it will harm the body in other ways. I'll explain later how to recognize when increased hair may be a sign of underlying hormonal disturbance. Usually hirsutism (the scientific term for excessive growth of hair) is not due to a serious disease, but it is important because of its tendency to cause embarrassment and social insecurity.

Some women who worry about facial and body hair have a normal amount but do not know it is normal. Women do their best to remove or otherwise conceal facial hair, and body hair is covered by clothes or shaved when shorts or bathing suits are worn. The results are so effective that each woman who successfully hides her own extra hair does not see any on the other women she knows, and therefore imagines she is the only one.

As a consequence of our culture's denial of normal female body-hair patterns, photographs of women rarely reveal any hair on their faces and bodies. Many famous women do have hair in these locations, but when they are photographed, techniques are used to make it nearly invisible. Usually the camera is slightly out of focus, a trick that is also effective in hiding wrinkles. If one looks very carefully at photographs of celebrities, however, facial hair can often be found. Many women who are embarrassed by their facial or body hair have no more than the stars who are held up as ideals of female beauty. I suspect that few things have contributed more to making women feel insecure about their appearance than the invention of photography that seems to show people as they really are but that actually alters their appearance.

Our culture's taboo about women's facial and body hair is so strong that the subject of hirsutism is not often discussed in women's magazines. This is surprising. Hirsutism is common enough that there must be more than a few female editors who are aware of the problem, because they have it themselves. Perhaps these editors also think they are the only ones with extra hair and do not realize how many of their readers have the same problem. The very success of women in concealing their hair makes everyone else unaware that there is any such problem. This lack of recognition extends to pharmaceutical company executives as well. When I have discussed the need for new drugs to be developed in this area, most have been unaware that such a problem existed.

Doctors and Hirsutism

Even doctors can fail to recognize hirsutism because their patients hide it and often are embarrassed to mention it. When I ask gynecologists or endocrinologists how many women they see with hirsutism, they often say only one or two a week. This is obviously wrong. A survey I have seen shows that one in ten women removes unwanted hair once a week or more. If we assume that the average doctor sees fifty to a hundred women in a typical week (probably an underestimate for many gynecologists), they should see at least ten hirsute women each week. They just aren't noticing. So far as I know, women doctors are not necessarily better than men at noticing increased body hair. Nurses may do better. They often spend more time with the patient, help her to undress, and pay more attention to matters of comfort and quality of life.

When I lecture to physicians and other health-care professionals, I spend considerable time teaching them how to recognize excessive hair after it has been bleached, shaved, or otherwise concealed. Unfortunately the problem among doctors may be not only lack of observation but one of attitude as well. It is a misconception to believe that if hair growth is not caused by a serious underlying disease or a severe hormonal disturbance that it is unimportant. Hair on your face and body looks the same whether your laboratory hormone measurements are abnormal or not. Hair in visible places is socially abnormal even if it is biologically normal. If it is bothersome and embarrassing, you have a right to have something done about it.

Doctors sometimes ask me how to tell if the amount of hair a woman has is abnormal. My answer is that I simply listen to the woman herself. If she takes the trouble to see a doctor, there is generally something there that she is legitimately concerned about and that merits evaluation and treatment. Among women I have seen who were concerned about hair growth, I can think of only a few who seemed to have no basis for their concern and were content with reassurance. If you are concerned about the quantity of face and body hair, you should know that this is as legitimate a concern as a fever, as irregular periods, as a lump in your breast. By this I do not mean that it is likely to be due to disease, but simply that it has as much right to be taken seriously.

More About Androgens

When I discussed androgens in Chapter Two, I emphasized the point that while they are sometimes called "male hormones," they are present normally in all women and account for some of the normal features of female development: appearance of underarm and pubic hair, as well as the increase in oiliness of the skin that is part of puberty. The levels women have, even when too high, are far lower than those in normal men. To be sure, some women do have androgen levels as high as men's, but this is quite rare and due to a specific endocrine disease. So even if you have an androgenic disorder, and even if you have been told that you have "too many male hormones," your androgen levels are not anywhere near those that men have.

There are several androgens. Testosterone is the most powerful. Most of it is carried in the blood, attached to a special protein called sex-hormone binding globulin (SHBG). Testosterone attached to this protein cannot move out of the blood into the tissues; SHBG serves as a reservoir of the hormone. Free testosterone is the dissolved form that is not attached to SHBG; it goes out of the blood into the tissues, including the target organs, such as the pilosebaceous unit. Free testosterone can be measured, but the measurement is more difficult than that for total testosterone; only a limited number of labs can perform it accurately. (It is also more expensive.) My own research has convinced me that free testosterone has a much closer relationship to androgenic problems in women than does the cruder measure of total testosterone. If you are being evaluated for an androgenic problem, I recommend that you request this test instead of only the total testosterone measurement. It is worth the extra cost.

Some of the effects of testosterone are due to the hormone itself, but others, especially hair loss, are more related to another form called DHT (dihydrotestosterone). DHT is made from testosterone in target tissues, including the pilosebaceous unit, by an enzyme called 5 alpha reductase. It is DHT levels in the skin that are important, so it is not useful to measure it in blood.

The other androgens that are helpful to measure if you have an androgenic disorder are androstenedione (ANDRO) and dehydroepiandrosterone sulfate (DHEA-S). Neither has much androgenic effect itself, but both can be converted into testosterone and so eventually contribute to androgenic changes. Knowing which gland is producing these hormones is important for both diagnosis and treatment. DHEA-S always comes from the adrenal gland, but testosterone and ANDRO can come from either the ovary or adrenal or both. How much comes from each is individual to each woman. Special testing called a dexamethasone suppression test can tell how much comes from each gland.

It may seem strange that sex hormones are made not only in the ovary (or testes, in the case of a man) but also in the adrenal gland. Most of what is important in female development and fertility does happen in the ovary. But the major hormones made in the adrenal are chemically similar to the androgens, so it is not surprising that the adrenal makes androgens also. In men, so much testosterone is made in the testicle that what is contributed by the adrenal is not important. But in women adrenal production contributes a significant amount.

Levels of all the androgens begin to rise as puberty begins; the appearance of pubic hair is the visible sign that this is happening. They continue to rise throughout the teens, plateau in the early twenties, and then gradually fall. Of course, some individuals have different patterns. However, as time goes on women are likely to have lower levels of free and total testosterone, androstenedione, and DHEA-S. When the ovary becomes quiescent with menopause, androgen levels fall further.

What Causes Some Women to Have Higher Androgen Levels?

It is time to describe the specific conditions that cause androgen levels to be high. I will discuss what can happen in the ovary and the adrenal gland separately, because even though the effects of the different conditions may be almost the same—acne, hirsutism, or alopecia can be caused by a problem in either the adrenal gland or the ovary—the underlying causes may be different. Treatments also differ somewhat, depending on whether the hormonal disturbance originates in the ovary or in the adrenal gland. My research on women with androgenic disorders shows that the adrenal gland is the primary source in somewhat over half of women with increased androgens.

Although slightly less common, ovarian androgen excess (often called polycystic ovary syndrome, or PCO) has gotten a disproportionate share of the attention. Ovarian androgen problems are more likely than adrenal ones to affect fertility, and this has been one reason for the emphasis on this form of androgenic disorder. One of the features of PCO is anovulation. Women with PCO may need medical help to get pregnant, whereas most with adrenal androgen excess ovulate and become pregnant without difficulty.

Adrenal androgenic disorders and the effects of PCO that are not related to fertility have also received less research attention. Not that research on infertility is not worthwhile. Many thousands of women with PCO who are now mothers would not have been without this research and the treatments it has discovered. But pregnancy is one part of a woman's life. The menstrual irregularity, hirsutism, acne, and hair loss that can be effects of PCO more often, unfortunately, go untreated.

ADRENAL ANDROGEN PROBLEMS

There are two kind of adrenal problems that can cause too much androgen to be secreted. The first is extremely common but oddly has no name. In this condition, the adrenal gland simply makes a little more androgen than it should. You may remember that in girls just before puberty begins to show, the adrenal gland starts to make more androgen than it did in childhood. This increase in adrenal androgen production is called adrenarche. In the many women with an androgenic disorder, this normal pubertal event seems to be a bit exaggerated. While all girls have this increase in androgen production in their adrenals, in a few the process goes a little too far; an androgenic disorder is the result. I call this condition exaggerated adrenarche. This choice of term emphasizes that it is not so much disease as a normal process that has gone a little too far.

The effects of exaggerated adrenarche are just what you see: severe or persistent acne, hirsutism, or androgenic alopecia. Testosterone or ANDRO or DHEA-S or a combination of them may be elevated, but more often are at the upper limit of normal. The dexamethasone suppression test, which I will explain later, clearly shows that the adrenal glands are the source of the androgens. Usually periods are normal, and it is rare for there to be any problem with fertility. In a few women, exaggerated adrenarche is more severe with higher androgen levels, and so, occasionally, this results in oligomenorrhea (infrequent periods).

The other causes of adrenal androgen excess are a group of conditions known as adrenal hyperplasia. Often they are called congenital adrenal hyperplasia, because at one time only forms detectable at birth were known. In such cases, development of the genitalia is affected. In the last decade, however, it has been discovered that the same conditions may have a later onset. What triggers the onset is not known. Adrenal hyperplasia tends to produce greater elevations of testosterone or other androgens than exaggerated adrenarche and is more likely to affect menstruation and fertility. There is great controversy about how common these late-onset forms of adrenal hyperplasia really are. One researcher has reported them in a high percentage of women with androgenic disorders; others, including myself, find them to be rarer. Some of this is due to population differences. Those of Ashkenazi Jewish and Inuit descent have a higher incidence than most other ethnic groups. Some preliminary work I did some years ago suggested that in a representative American population, only a small percentage of women with androgenic disorders have any form of adrenal hyperplasia.

The cause of adrenal hyperplasia is an enzyme blockage that causes the adrenal gland to make its hormones in incorrect proportions. The exact pattern of hormone excess depends on the particular forms of adrenal hyperplasia. In some forms, mineralocorticoids are overproduced, and high blood pressure can result.

OVARIAN ANDROGEN PROBLEMS

I started with adrenal androgen problems because they are both more common and simpler to understand. But ovarian problems are almost as common and have another effect: anovulation, or lack of production of eggs. In this situation (see Chapter Four), the pituitary gland and the ovary do not interact normally. As a result, follicles start to mature at the beginning of the cycle but are unable to proceed to actual ovulation. Over time, more and more follicles accumulate in this condition of thwarted development and give the ovary a characteristic appearance known as polycystic. The capsule, the outer lining of the ovary, becomes thickened as well. This thick capsule seems to be one of the factors inhibiting ovulation, because it makes it harder for ova to get out of the ovary. This condition begins in the teens, but it may be some time before enough follicles accumulate to give the ovary the polycystic appearance. When follicles fail to mature, they remain in the ovary and continue to make hormones. When a woman has polycystic ovary syndrome (PCO), her follicles have increased numbers of theca cells, which make androgens. Normal ovaries have theca cells, but not nearly so many.

Modern treatment for ovarian androgen problems is hormonal, replacing surgery. An old operation, ovarian wedge resection, produced temporary benefit but is outmoded. The term polycystic ovary refers to the appearance or anatomy of the ovary. In PCO, the ovary contains many cysts. For most lay people, the word "cyst" suggests a tumor or something that might turn into one. Actually "cyst" comes from the Greek word meaning bladder and merely refers to any fluid-filled structure. Most cysts are not tumors at all; they are benign and do not pose problems. This is the case with the tiny cysts in polycystic ovaries. (True tumors may contain some fluid and therefore be cystic. How to tell whether a particular cyst is a tumor or not is beyond the scope of this book. The message here is that a cyst is not always something to be worried about.)

I have seen some women who were told they had polycystic ovaries and were frightened by the word cyst, thinking it meant that they had an ovarian tumor. Some have still been worried, years later. There is no need for this, and so I avoid using the term "polycystic ovaries" as much as possible. I prefer to refer to the condition as ovarian androgen excess. This is more accurate as well, because not all women whose condition fits the usual hormonal criteria for PCO actually have cysts in their ovaries. And some women who have many cysts in their ovaries do not have the hormonal problems that go with PCO.

There has been much and needless confusion about PCO. The term PCO refers to a change in the *appearance* of the ovary. But what is really important to the woman who has PCO is how her ovary *functions*. A woman is usually considered to have PCO if she has a high androgen level and oligomenorrhea or amenorrhea (no menstrual flow). Neither of these criteria has to do with how the ovary looks. In fact, PCO is probably not one but several different diseases with slightly different characteristics. In some forms, the ovary has the classical polycystic appearance, but in others it does not. Some women whose ovaries look polycystic have normal periods, no problem with hirsutism, and they ovulate every month. So whether the ovary is polycystic or not can be a red herring.

In the early puberty of normal girls, the ovary goes through a stage when it looks mildly polycystic. Sometimes an ultrasound scan is done for an unrelated reason (pelvic pain, for example), and parents are told that their daughter has polycystic ovaries, when in fact her ovaries are going through a normal developmental stage.

Many worries could be avoided if the term "polycystic ovaries" were to be dropped from our medical language. Unfortunately the term is so familiar that I am sure it will not be.

There are several theories about the cause of PCO, but

none are proven. One factor is that the pituitary gland secretes luteinizing hormone (LH) in the wrong rhythm. Another is that it is caused by the action of local hormones within the ovary itself. So far, none of these theories has been completely proven. Fortunately we do have a good understanding of how to diagnose and treat ovarian androgen excess.

ANDROGEN-PRODUCING TUMORS

Tumors are a common cause of worry but an uncommon cause of androgen excess. Textbooks necessarily give emphasis to the most serious conditions, so if you look up hirsutism or androgen excess in an endocrinology text, you may find lengthy discussions of adrenal and ovarian tumors and cancers. These do happen, but not very often. In my patient population of 3,000 women with androgenic disorders, less than ten had a tumor of the ovary or the adrenal gland. I occasionally get calls from other physicians, asking about patients of theirs with elevated androgens and wondering if a tumor is a possibility. Almost invariably this possibility is a false alarm. Perhaps this excessive fear of tumors is due to an unconscious—and mistaken—assumption that testosterone does not belong in a woman's body.

Androgens and Female Sexual Orientation

Though they rarely ask about it, I suspect some of the women I see worry about what having high androgen levels means for their sexuality and gender identity. I can summarize my fifteen years of experience with androgen disorders by saying that androgens appear to have no effect whatever on either. Some of my patients describe very active sex lives with many different partners; others have been virgins with no evident interest in forming a sexual relationship of any kind. And there has been everything in between, with the majority having monogamous relationships. A number of my patients have told me that they are lesbians. Their feelings about their excessive hair are the same as those of the other women I see. Women with androgenic disorders are a cross-section of American women who just happen to have problems with acne, increased facial hair, alopecia, or their menstrual cycles.

Although, at first thought, it might seem that more androgens might give a woman a more male-like sexuality, this is clearly not the case. Certainly no one changes erotic preference because her androgens go up. And it should be kept in mind that even women with elevated testosterone levels still have amounts far less than those in men. Prenatal exposure to very high androgen levels, an exceedingly rare event, may have some effects on gender development. There is no lack of theories in this area, but the data are difficult to interpret, so no clear conclusion is possible now.

Androgenic Disorders, Stress, and Weight Gain

Two common concerns women have about hormonal problems are their relationship to stress and their influence on weight. The idea that stress is a major cause of illness is a popular one, and is sometimes valid. Acne and alopecia, in particular, are likely to be attributed to stress. Acne begins in the teens, which for most people is when stress begins to be a conscious factor in their lives. An expression for saying one is under great stress is to say it is "making my hair fall out." However, there is no evidence whatsoever that stress causes androgenic disorders, though it may make them harder to live with. It is true that the adrenal gland is one of the organs involved in the body's protective response to stress, but stress does not seem to have much effect on androgen levels; it is other adrenal hormones that are affected by stress. Blaming stress for a condition is itself stressful, because often there is nothing you can do to stop being stressed. Self-blame is unnecessary; stress won't give you acne or make your hair fall out.

The relationship of androgenic disorders to becoming overweight is more complex. The average weight of women with hirsutism is higher than the overall female population. This is not true of acne and alopecia patients in my studies. Heavier women seem to have more marked androgen excess. They are more likely to have oligomenorrhea or amenorrhea and to have cholesterol problems. Some endocrinologists believe that becoming obese sets off PCO in certain women, and this is entirely possible. Obesity causes insulin levels to be higher, and insulin can stimulate the ovaries to make more androgens. There is another theory that androgenic disorders cause weight gain because of the anabolic (metabolism stimulating) effect of androgens. This is not the whole story, because some women with high androgens are slender. However, it is possible that some women may be susceptible to an anabolic or appetite-increasing effect of androgens. Unfortunately lowering the androgens does not make weight come off by itself.

Laboratory Tests for Androgenic Disorders

Medicine now emphasizes lab tests, probably more than it should. Yet there is no doubt that in endocrinology our ability to understand why someone is having the problem she is and what can be done about it is in no small part due to the advances in laboratory diagnosis. Below I list specific tests and what they can tell you about the cause of your problem. This section will mainly be of interest to readers who have had the test discussed and want an in-depth account of what it means. I suggest you read about testosterone and the dexamethasone suppression test, but you can skip the other sections if they do not pertain to you.

TESTOSTERONE

I've already mentioned that there are separate measurements for the testosterone that is bound to sex-hormone binding globulin (SHBG) and that which is free. As its name implies, the total testosterone test measures all of the testosterone. The free portion is only 1 or 2 percent of the total, and so is more difficult to measure.

Both forms of testosterone affect the body. Free testosterone does so most directly since, as I said earlier, it can move most quickly into the tissues. But the bound testosterone is gradually released by the SHBG and becomes free testosterone, which in turn finds its way out of the blood and into the skin and other tissues. If either form is elevated, it is significant. In mild situations, free testosterone is more likely to be elevated. But sometimes free testosterone is normal and total testosterone is high. Both mean there is increased testosterone.

Some women with androgen problems have normal testosterone levels. There are several reasons for this. First, the levels fluctuate; by chance, blood may have been taken when the levels happen to be at their lowest. Second, there is a strong tendency for androgen levels to go down with age. Testosterone—and all the other androgens—are at their highest in the late teens or very early twenties, and they work their way down after that. However, once the hair follicles have been stimulated by higher levels of testosterone, they tend to stay active. High androgens program the hair follicle to be more active indefinitely.

What causes some women with increased androgens to have

acne and not hirsutism? The answer lies in the response of a woman's skin to testosterone. Whether she will have acne or increased hair growth or both is explained by skin differences rather than by hormonal differences. The point of testing is to find the underlying hormonal factors, because it is these that determine what will be the most effective treatment. Treatment depends as much on the underlying hormone change as on the skin problem. Often the hormonal part of the treatments for hirsutism and for acne will be the same.

A few years ago a test called 3 alpha diol G was introduced; it was intended to measure one form of skin sensitivity to testosterone. Despite strong claims by its inventors, many endocrinologists, including myself, have not found it to match well at all with a woman's hair growth.

I have emphasized that free testosterone, which always includes the measurement of total testosterone, is a more relevant test than that for total testosterone by itself. What if you had a workup and only total testosterone was done? Does this mean you have to have a test for free testosterone now? Not necessarily. But even if your total testosterone was normal, there is always the possibility that the free value would be elevated. Whoever interprets the test should keep this in mind. Especially when total testosterone is at a high normal level, free testosterone is often slightly elevated.

So far, I've talked about normal and mildly elevated testosterone levels, but not yet about very high values. Fortunately these are very rare in women. An androgen-secreting tumor has to be considered if your testosterone level is over about 150 ng/dl.

The two glands in which testosterone-secreting tumors can occur are, as you might expect, the ovary and the adrenal gland. If you have very high testosterone, be sure you are being cared for by someone with real expertise in this area, because the selection and interpretation of the tests can be quite complicated. Generally they consist of measurements of other hormones, a dexamethasone suppression test, and imaging studies of the ovary and the adrenal gland. Ultrasound is best for the ovary, and CT for the adrenal gland.

Other factors that raise the possibility of a tumor are symptoms that come on suddenly and increase rapidly, or that are severe. Most hirsutism and acne develop gradually. A woman who had no problem with hair growth and suddenly develops a lot of it needs to have this evaluated promptly. The very high levels of androgens found in tumors can also produce changes that are more extreme, such as deepening of the voice or actual balding, not just mild alopecia. I remember a young woman who had a testosterone-producing tumor that was discovered because, in addition to a marked increase in facial hair, she could no longer hit the high notes that she'd been able to sing before. I am sure that ten times as many women with androgen problems worry that they have a tumor as actually have one. If you have signs suggesting a tumor, testing can determine with certainty if you do or not. If your ovarian ultrasound and adrenal CT are normal, you can stop worrying.

Some women have high testosterone levels (over 150 ng/dl), but no tumor is found. They generally have either marked polycystic ovaries (hyperthecosis) or adrenal hyperplasia. Both conditions can be treated. Testosterone levels this high are likely to cause problems and definitely need thorough diagnosis and effective treatment.

ANDROSTENEDIONE

I have emphasized testosterone because it is the most important androgen. However, it is also useful to know what your androstenedione level is, because high levels also contribute to androgen-related problems. Normal levels are up to about 250 ng/dl. If your level is higher, you will need a dexamethasone suppression test (see below) to find out if it is coming from your ovary or your adrenal gland.

DHEA-S

Like androstenedione, this substance can be made into testosterone. DHEA-S stands for dehydroepiandrosterone sulfate, but no one ever refers to it by this cumbersome name. DHEA-S does not act in your body like an androgen unless the level is very high—over 450 or 500 mcg/dl. A level over 700 mcg/dl raises concern of a possible tumor. I need to point out a source of confusion about DHEA-S measurements. For some reason, different laboratories select different units when reporting DHEA-S levels. For example, what I have called 300 mcg/dl might also be called 3 mcg/ml or 3,000 ng/ml. So don't panic because I told you a level above 700 mcg/dl is of concern, and you just found out that yours is 4,000 ng/ml; this is just 400 mcg/dl. Look at the lab slip, which will tell you the normal range for the units it is using.

DEXAMETHASONE SUPPRESSION TEST

This is a very useful and important test. It is not done very commonly, and when it is, it is not always done correctly. In medical jargon, the detailed and precise instructions as to how a test is to be done is called a protocol. Protocols include doses of medication and exact timing of when blood samples are to be drawn.

The dexamethasone suppression test—or, more simply, "dex test"—belongs to a family known in endocrinology as dynamic tests. These are an active method of diagnosis. Instead of simply taking blood and seeing what the hormone level happens to be, dynamic tests look at the way the body's hormonal system responds to certain stimuli. The dex test is a suppression test. The concept of suppression is a very important one for understanding how androgenic disorders are treated. When dexamethasone is given, the pituitary gland responds by decreasing its secretion of ACTH (adrenocorticotropin); therefore the adrenal is suppressed. When suppressed, a gland stops making its hormones. In the case of the adrenal gland, this means that levels of glucocorticoids and androgens go down. In some conditions, the adrenal or other gland will no longer obey the pituitary's control signals, and a suppression test can reveal this situation.

In androgenic disorders, the dex test is used to find out how much of a woman's androgens are coming from her adrenals and how much from her ovaries. Because the adrenals are suppressed by the dexamethasone, whatever androgens appear in the blood must have come from the ovary. For example, if you had a testosterone level of 80 ng/dl before taking the dexamethasone and 40 afterward, half of your testosterone would be coming from your adrenals and half from your ovaries. If, on the other hand, your testosterone did not fall at all, then you could conclude that all of it is coming from your ovaries. A third case would be that your testosterone dropped very low—say to 15 ng/dl; then the interpretation would be that nearly all of it is coming from your adrenal gland. The important point is that the dex test can tell which glands your androgens are coming from; this may have practical use in helping to choose the treatment most likely to be effective.

There are two different kinds of protocols for the dex test. In some, dexamethasone is given for two days or less. This will suppress glucocorticoids but not androgens, which take five or more days to suppress. Sometimes this shorter dex test is given to women to test where their androgens are coming from. When this is done, the adrenal gland is not fully suppressed, and the ovary may be blamed for making androgens that are actually coming from the adrenal gland. In some of the early research on the question of the relative roles of the adrenal gland and ovary in making androgens, this mistake was made. The dexamethasone was given for only two days; the result was overestimation of how much testosterone comes from the ovaries. Unfortunately this misinformation was never formally corrected and is still found in some textbooks.

If you have a dex test, be sure it uses a protocol that is proper for finding out about androgens. The one I use for my patients is to take dexamethasone in a dose of 0.375 mg four times a day for eight to ten days. This dose is one and a half of the smallest-size tablets. Whichever of your androgens were elevated are measured before you start the dexamethasone and again at the end of the course. It is essential to take the medication right up until the blood is drawn for the second set of tests. A few women notice some restlessness on this dose, but there are rarely other side effects because the dex is given for a relatively short time. This dose would be too high for long-term treatment.

Sometimes it is assumed that, if the DHEA-S is elevated, the problem is in the adrenal gland. My research has clearly shown that this is not true. The only way to determine if testosterone or ANDRO is coming from the adrenal is to do a dex test. It is useful enough to be well worth the inconvenience. Not every women with facial hair or acne or other androgen-related problem needs a dex test. If your testosterone and other androgens are normal, it is unnecessary. In that case, both your ovaries and your adrenal glands are functioning normally, and the problem is the sensitivity of your skin to normal levels of androgens.

SHBG (SEX-HORMONE BINDING GLOBULIN)

This special protein is made in the liver and circulates in the blood. Its function is to bind testosterone and estrogen so that they will not go into the tissues too rapidly. The levels are higher in women because estrogen acts on the liver to stimulate it to make SHBG. Androgens have the opposite effect; they lower SHBG levels, and so men have less. Because SHBG normally acts as a sponge, sopping up androgens, a lack of SHBG tends to mean that more androgen gets into the tissues. The way estrogen counteracts androgen is by raising SHBG to slow the leakage of androgen into the skin and other tissues. If your SHBG is low, the testosterone in your blood will affect your body more.

LH/FSH RATIO

This is just the calculated ratio of the two pituitary hormones that control the ovary. There is an old idea that in polycystic ovary syndrome (PCO) this ratio will be 3 or higher. My own research shows this to be untrue. The FSH/LH ratio does not tell whether your androgens are coming from your ovary or your adrenal gland. Measuring LH and FSH is sometimes helpful, but much less so than measuring the androgens themselves or doing a dexamethasone suppression test. The LH/FSH ratio has not turned out to be as useful as originally thought.

PROLACTIN

This is the pituitary hormone that makes it possible for the breast to make milk. High levels suppress the ovary, as has been discussed in Chapter Four. Some studies have shown that prolactin is sometimes higher in androgenic disorders, especially polycystic ovary syndrome. However, although the levels are higher, the difference is slight, still within the normal range. If you have a high prolactin level, do not blame it on an androgenic disorder. You will need tests to see if you have a pituitary problem. Some women have both an androgenic disorder and a pituitary prolactin problem. Both are common and, by coincidence, some women get both.

SPECIAL STEROID HORMONE MEASUREMENTS

Steroid hormones are made in a woman's ovary and adrenal glands in a long series of steps. At each step a particular chemical is formed which is usually not measured. However, if there is a genetic problem with the system of enzymes that make the hormones, levels of these earlier forms go up. Measurement of some of these hormone precursors is used to diagnose adrenal hyperplasia, a group of conditions I described earlier in this chapter. The enzyme 17 hydroxyprogesterone is used to diagnose 21 hydroxylase deficiency; 17 hydroxypregnenolone, for 3 beta hydroxysteroid dehydrogenase deficiency (3 beta HSD); and 11 deoxycortisol (compound S), for 11 hydroxylase deficiency. I mention all these for the sake of completeness and in case you hear the terms. The conditions are rare and their diagnoses rather technical, so I will not describe them in detail here. Treatment, however, is straightforward and the same as for other forms of adrenal androgen excess, described in Chapter Seven.

ACTH STIMULATION TEST

This is the opposite of the dexamethasone suppression test in that it tries to stimulate the adrenal gland instead of suppressing it. It is used for the diagnosis of the various forms adrenal hyperplasia. An injection of ACTH (adrenocortico-tropin, the pituitary hormone which controls the adrenal) produces a much greater than normal rise in the substances I mentioned in the preceding paragraph, and the diagnosis can be confirmed. This test is also used to diagnose underactivity of the adrenal gland. In Addison's disease, for example, the adrenal gland has been destroyed by the immune system, and levels of cortisol (or androgens) cannot rise in response to ACTH.

URINARY FREE CORTISOL

There is another group of conditions in which the adrenal gland makes too much of its main hormone, cortisol. The best way to test for this is to measure cortisol in a twenty-four-hour urine collection. Because its levels vary in the blood every few minutes, a single random measurement of cortisol is not very helpful. Even when blood is drawn at two different times of day, the so-called "AM-PM cortisol," blood levels of cortisol are not very helpful.

Because signs of too much cortisol (Cushing syndrome) include weight gain, acne, and the stopping of periods, it is sometimes necessary to distinguish it from the far more common female androgenic disorders. Cushing's syndrome is usually a more serious disease; if there is any chance of it being present, it is important to test for it.

Collecting a twenty-four-hour urine sample is simple, if not always convenient. The lab will supply a proper container. For some tests this has a special preservative in it, so be sure to use the container you were given. Empty your bladder when you wake up in the morning, as you normally would, then save the urine from all subsequent voidings, up to and including the first one the next morning. If you forget to save one voiding, you may need to start all over again the next morning. The container with the urine should be stored in the refrigerator.

* * *

This chapter has described how androgens can have unwanted effects on a woman's body and how these androgenic disorders can be diagnosed. The next chapter will explain what can be done to treat these conditions.

Chapter Six

•

Androgenic Disorders Can Be Treated

*A*ndrogenic disorders affect almost one out of ten American women, but they can, in most cases, be safely and effectively treated. In my experience, most women who have an androgenic disorder want to be relieved of the unpleasant changes it produces. However, some are hesitant, either because they feel guilty about being concerned with their appearance or because they have been given misinformation about the effectiveness or safety of treatment. Misinformation may have come from friends, or even from physicians who are opposed to treatment of a problem that mainly affects appearance.

Physicians who believe that appearance problems are too trivial to merit diagnosis and treatment usually consider themselves to have risen above what they regard as superficial concerns. More likely, however, they are just sharing the general cultural hypocrisy about these matters. I doubt that they would be as unconcerned with their own, or a friend's or a family member's appearance. I am not suggesting that treatment for appearance problems should be entered into casually. The same care needs to be taken by doctor and patient as should be taken for any decision to use medication. I am saying that it is as legitimate to be treated for extra hair growth or acne or alopecia as it is to be treated for headaches, high blood pressure, or the flu.

There is nothing inherently wrong with taking medications to look better. Note that the issue is not taking medications to improve on nature, but to restore your skin and hair to how they should normally look. At the same time, correcting an appearance problem should not involve taking medications that are likely to be hazardous or that carry risks of serious side effects. There is nothing wrong with taking medicine to clear acne, to decrease facial hair, or to stop scalp hair from thinning. There is a lot wrong with taking dangerous medicines for these conditions. No matter how desperate you feel about a change in your appearance, the use of dangerous drugs is not justified. Drugs used to treat androgenic disorders generally must be taken for a long time, usually years rather than weeks or months. It is better not to start a treatment unless it is safe to take it for the long term.

Fortunately the medications that are effective in helping androgenic disorders are safe if properly used and monitored. They can have side effects, of course, but these tend to be inconvenient or mildly uncomfortable rather than truly harmful. The side effects are reversible; that is, they go away when the medication is stopped. Of course, you will need to know about potential adverse effects, as well as benefits, in order to decide between your various options, and I will spell out possible problems with each treatment in detail. Some medications used for androgenic disorders are not as safe as others; I will alert you to them. But the message of this chapter is, I believe, one of the most optimistic of the book: If you have an androgenic disorder, there is safe and effective treatment for you.

Principles of Treatment
of Androgenic Disorders

Women are not all the same. As I have stressed, different women who seem to have the same skin or hair problem may have quite different underlying hormonal factors causing it. Furthermore, each woman has other aspects of her hormonal situation that must be considered in designing the treatment that will have the best chance of working out for her. To be right for you, a treatment must not only take away the problem; it must not cause other problems nor interfere with your life.

Whenever possible, I have the women who consult me return after their first visit (which has consisted of discussion, a very detailed physical examination, and testing) to discuss the treatment and plan it on an individual basis. Taking enough time to properly plan will usually result in time saved in the long run, because the treatment will be more suited to your needs. If you are contemplating treatment for an androgenic disorder, I recommend you give yourself the time to study the different choices, so that when you do make your decision, it will be the right one for you.

There are two major factors in all androgenic problems: the levels of the androgens themselves and the body's sensitivity to the androgens. Treatments can alter both factors. Some lower the levels of androgens; others block their effect on the skin or hair. Methods of treatment that lower hormones are called suppression methods. Medications that block the action of androgens are called anti-androgens or androgen antagonists. These, in effect, desensitize the oil gland or hair follicle by filling up the hormone receptors so that androgens have no place to attach.

Testing can determine the relative contributions of high hormone levels and skin sensitivity. It can also determine which hormones are causing the problems, and the extent to which they come from the ovary or the adrenal gland.

To see how the information gleaned from lab tests is used to devise treatments capable of clearing acne, decreasing facial and body hair, and protecting scalp hair, let us return to the stories of some of the women I have told you about in earlier chapters.

How Increased Hair Growth Is Treated

Sharon, you may remember, had enough facial hair that she would not go out in the morning until she had removed it with a razor. By mid-afternoon she had to reapply makeup to conceal the dark color of the returning hairs. Her testosterone was mildly elevated at 85 ng/dl, and the dex test showed that virtually all of it was coming from her ovary. Ellen, on the other hand, also had excessive hair growth, though not so much that she had to use a razor every morning. Plucking and bleaching worked for her, though she wanted less hair. Her testosterone level was normal at 46 ng/dl. A third woman, Lenore, had acne rather than excessive hair, but her underlying hormonal problem was similar to Sharon's and Ellen's: increased action of androgens on her pilosebaceous unit. Lenore's testosterone was elevated, but the source was different from Sharon's; most was coming from her adrenal gland. Lenore's skin responded by making too much oil rather than too much hair.

Ellen's hormonal pattern was simplest. Her androgens were all normal, so there was no need for her even to have a dex test. Her problem was simply skin sensitivity to androgens. Treatment for this is straightforward: use of an anti-androgen. The one I suggested for her was spironolactone, the most generally used for this purpose. For Sharon, I also recommended spironolactone but added the oral contraceptive OrthoCyclen® (OrthoPharmaceutical Corp.) in order to suppress the activity of her ovaries, which were the source of the slightly increased amounts of testosterone in her blood. The pill also served to regulate her cycle and protect her uterus from the effects of anovulation.

Lenore also started on spironolactone to block the action of the androgens on her skin, but she also began dexamethasone in a very low dose, to decrease the activity of her adrenal glands, which were the source of her slightly excessive amounts of testosterone.

Neither Sharon nor Lenore had any side effects from their medications. Ellen did have the side effect from spironolactone that is most annoying: It made her periods come too close together. Sometimes this straightens itself out after two or three months, but in Ellen's case it did not. As she put it, "I don't like getting it once a month, but I never really imagined I'd have to have it even more often." We agreed she would also use an oral contraceptive to take advantage of its ability to regulate the menstrual cycle. The very next month her periods returned to their familiar four-weekly pattern.

How well did treatment work for these three women, and what other sorts of problems did they have with treatment?

Sharon first noticed a change when she had been on treatment for between three and four months. In the morning when she first looked in the mirror, the hair growing back was not quite as long, though it was just as thick and dark. But nine months after starting treatment, when she came for her next follow-up, Sharon reported that she had begun to see more improvement. Her facial hair was lighter and thinner. And it was definitely not as long when she removed it each morning. While she still freshened her makeup each afternoon, she felt less anxiety about the problem. She no longer worried if she had to stay in a meeting past 2:30.

I have now been treating Sharon for three years, and she has shown steady improvement. It is not that all the extra hair is gone. In fact, Sharon still uses a razor each morning. But she told me this about the benefits of treatment: "It's changed my life completely. Sure, I don't like using a razor every morning; that part may not be much different. But once I've done that, I feel secure for the first time since my teens. I don't have to fear that if anyone looks at me closely they'll be surprised to see a beard. I've always felt like a woman, but now I look like one, too. That old lack of confidence is just gone." Nor does Sharon now have to go home to remove hair before she can go out for the evening. Of course, we both wish there were no trace of extra hair; for women with very heavy growth of facial hair, this is not always possible. But the change, as Sharon's own words reveal, is sufficient for her to feel normal, something she did not feel before treatment.

One reason some doctors think hirsutism treatment doesn't work is that they regard a result in which not all the hair is gone as a failure. They do not recognize that even a limited result is far preferable to life with constant insecurity that the embarrassing secret will be revealed.

Hair growth is something that changes slowly, and any treatment takes a long time to work. It is not so much the medications as the processes they are acting on that require so much time. This can be very frustrating for a problem you must face every morning in the mirror. If you are being treated for hirsutism, promise yourself to be patient.

Ellen had a milder degree of hirsutism due to hair follicle sensitivity; she did not have any hormonal disorder. Spironolactone was her only medication. But her time to respond was similar to Sharon's. At four months, her first visit to me after starting treatment, she told me with some disappointment that she had not noticed any change. But when I asked if it took her as long to pluck out hairs each morning, she thought and admitted that there were possibly fewer each morning than she'd had before. Like Sharon, she thought that the hairs were not thinner or lighter at this point. When hirsutism is treated, the first change is that the hair grows out more slowly; this can be noticed in three or four months. Treatment eventually causes the hair to become finer in diameter, softer to the touch, and lighter in color, but these changes do not begin to be noticeable until sometime in the second six months of treatment. Hair continues to become progressively lighter and thinner during the next year or two of treatment. The area of skin covered with hair often decreases also, especially on the lower abdomen, thighs, forearm, and chest, as well as on the cheeks. This also is a gradual change that may take a year or more. Is it worth it to wait so long for the hair to lighten and decrease? For women who have been willing to try the treatments, it definitely has been.

Let's go back to Ellen. Once I drew her attention to it, she realized there had been some initial signs of improvement at four months. Her patience was rewarded when, six more months into her treatment, she found that there was a very definite decrease in the amount of hair. It was lighter and finer, and there was less of it. There was further improvement over the following months, so that she was now comfortable wearing a two-piece bathing suit, something she would not have considered before because of the dark hair on her upper thighs and abdomen.

There is considerable variation in the degree to which excessive hair decreases with treatment. For some women, like Ellen, the extra hair seems to virtually disappear. For others, like Sharon, there may be almost as much hair, but it becomes so much finer and lighter so that it can be effectively concealed. Most women I treat end up with a result somewhere in between. They have much less hair and that which remains is less visible, but some still needs to be removed. Because the chin and upper lip as well as the area around the areolae and the line between navel and pubis are very sensitive to androgens, some hairs are likely to remain in these locations. Indeed, many women who do not consider themselves to have excessive hair have it on these places.

The majority of women with hirsutism can get an excellent result from treatment, but it must be the proper treatment. More than one medication is often required. One is almost always an androgen blocker, such as spironolactone or flutamide. Birth control pills or dexamethasone may be important as adjuncts, but they usually cannot decrease hair growth very much by themselves. I feel it is very important in explaining any medical treatment not to exaggerate the benefits or to soft-peddle the side effects. You need accurate information to be able to make medical decisions that you will be satisfied with.

Realistic expectations are necessary. Mild hirsutism may go away almost completely. Some body and facial hair will be left, but no more than the usual amount for other women. Ellen's story is representative of how mild hirsutism responds to treatment. More marked hirsutism usually does not disappear completely. Frequent removal may still be necessary, but it will give a much better result. As Sharon's story shows, this change may make a major difference in your life if you have this degree of increased hair. With only occasional exceptions, women treated for hirsutism experience significant improvement.

A good way for me to give you a further idea of what endocrine treatment for hair-growth problems can accomplish is to return to the story of another of my patients.

Keisha had fewer hairs than Sharon, but they were just as thick and noticeable. In addition, her hairs were curly and, when they grew back after plucking, tended to get caught under the skin and become infected. Black skin tends to show scarring more because it has more pigmentation. Dark Caucasians and Asians also show more of this post-inflammatory hyperpigmentation than those who are fair-skinned.

Keisha had been plucking hairs as her method of removal.

This is the most common method used by women because it is easy and effective. It is not really a good method, however, because each time a hair is pulled out the skin is traumatized; eventually scarring and hyperpigmentation occur. Repeated plucking from the chin produces an irregular, lumpy appearance. I explained all this to Keisha and suggested that while she was waiting for the medication to work, she use a depilatory cream and avoid plucking. Depilatories do not remove the hair under the skin and so are less likely to result in ingrown hair problems. Keisha's laboratory results were similar to Sharon's, except that her testosterone level was slightly higher. Her treatment was the same: spironolactone and the oral contraceptive OrthoCyclen®. Keisha's improvement took several months to show itself, just as Sharon's and Ellen's did. Over time, the hairs became thinner, and there were fewer of them. And there was another change that was perhaps the most important for her: because her facial hairs were now softer, the problem of hairs becoming ingrown and infected went away. The darkening of her skin in the old scar areas did not completely go away over a year and a half, but it became much lighter and less noticeable so that it could now be completely concealed with makeup.

All of the women I have been telling you about were well into adulthood. While it is possible to help hirsutism that has been present for decades, starting treatment early gives the best result. Early treatment is also better psychologically; it is better to decrease the hair growth before it has caused serious social embarrassment.

Endocrine Treatment of Acne

Lenore's treatment was different from that of the other women I've mentioned because it included suppression of her adrenal gland with dexamethasone. This had nothing to do with the fact that she had acne rather than hirsutism. Endocrine treatment depends on the underlying hormone pattern rather than on the particular skin change. Unlike Lenore, Ellen had a change in her menstrual cycle with spironolactone, a problem which was solved by the addiction of an oral contraceptive. Side effects can happen whichever problem someone is being treated for.

Lenore did not have to wait very long to see improvement. Within a month, she noticed that her skin was much less oily. Some of the old cysts were still present, although they were getting smaller as they gradually healed; this process can, unfortunately, take months. I had suggested to Lenore that she continue to take an antibiotic. She had been reluctant to because, as she put it, "I think I've been on all the antibiotics there are, and they've never done anything for me. Even if they seem to work for a while, the zits always come back." Lenore had tried all three antibiotics usually prescribed for acne: tetracycline, minocycline, and erythromycin. The first had given her yeast infections, the second was extremely expensive, and the third upset her stomach.

My recommendation was to go back on erythromycin in a dose of 500 mg twice a day (an equivalent is E-Mycin® [Boots] 333 mg twice a day). This dose, about half that used for acute infections such as strep throat, rarely causes upset stomach and does not have the tendency to cause photosensitivity or vaginal yeast infections, which are problems with tetracycline.

Why did I suggest going back on a medication that had not worked before? Simply because an antibiotic will speed up healing of the existing lesions, something hormonal treatment will not do. Hormonal treatment stops the lesions from coming out, but it does not help them to heal after they have appeared, whereas antibiotics do. Hormonal therapy will work without antibiotics, but it will take longer.

There are two steps in acne therapy. The first is to get the skin to clear up; this sometimes requires several medications, which work at different steps in the acne process. The second, when the skin has been really clear for at least several months, is to minimize the amount of medication. Lenore's acne would still have healed without the erythromycin, but it would have taken longer. People with acne want it to go away as soon as possible.

Lenore had noticed the decrease in the oiliness of her skin within the first month; as her cysts gradually healed, she noticed that there were fewer new ones, but that she did have occasional papules (raised red bumps without any pus in them). By four months, even these had stopped coming out, and her skin was almost clear. Her next visit was nine months after starting the medications. When I walked into the exam room, I almost thought I had the wrong chart. Here was a young women with a peaches and cream complexion. Not only were there no active lesions (though Lenore did say that she had an occasional small whitehead); the scarring had become nearly invisible. Hormonal treatment does not in itself alter scars, but because the chronic inflammation stops, the skin smoothes out and pits become shallower and much less noticeable. "I wish I had found out about this five years ago" was how Lenore summarized her feelings about the treatment. Hormonal treatment of acne can be dramatically successful. It gives a better result than other approaches because it works at the cause: the hormonally stimulated excessive oil production.

A very few women do not respond to endocrine treatment for acne, though it is unclear why. I see this lack of response very rarely, less than 5 percent of the time. Nearly all the women who come to an endocrinologist because of acne have seen several other doctors first, so it is the most difficult cases that I see. Yet it is very rare for endocrine treatment not to work.

Hormonal Treatment for Extra Hair and Acne: The Details About the Anti-androgens

The principle behind anti-androgens (also called androgen antagonists) is straightforward. Androgens act on receptors within the cell to cause them to attach to the DNA and thereby alter gene activity. An otherwise less active gene then steps up its activity. The result might be more sebum production or increased metabolism in the hair follicle, which eventually leads to darker, thicker hairs. Anti-androgens and other hormone antagonists also bind to the receptor, but because they are not identical to the actual hormone they do not activate the receptor, but just sit there on it. This effectively keeps the real hormone from moving onto the receptor and activating it. The result is a decrease in the effect of that hormone on the body.

Almost always, hormone blockade is less than 100 percent. Unless extremely large amounts are given, not all the receptors are filled with hormone blocker, and some real hormone finds its way to receptors. Some hormone effect occurs, although much less than without the antagonist. The result is that while anti-androgens work, they do not always completely take the problem away; rather they ameliorate it.

If hormone levels are high, more of the molecules can beat the molecules of the antagonist to the receptor and the antagonist will have less effect. When androgen levels are high, an antagonist will work better with other medication to suppress the gland producing the excessive androgens. This is why Sharon needed birth control pills in addition to the anti-androgen spironolactone. The mildly excessive amount of testosterone coming from her ovaries was suppressed by the birth control pills. Lenore also had elevated testosterone, but since that came from her adrenals, a different medication, dexamethasone, was used. The principle, however, was the same:

to lower the amount of testosterone in the blood so that the androgen blocker would be more effective. Ellen simply had skin that was very sensitive to androgens; her testosterone and other androgens were normal. Hers is the most common situation in women with androgenic skin or hair problems. Only anti-androgens are needed, although some women also take the pill for contraception or for irregular periods.

In general, androgenic skin conditions require an anti-androgen to improve. Some women with acne will improve on the pill or dexamethasone alone, but women with hirsutism or androgenic alopecia rarely are helped by these medications alone. Even when acne responds to the pill, the skin often clears even more if an anti-androgen is also taken.

The function of androgens in women is unclear. They are necessary for pubic and underarm hair to form, and they probably play an anabolic role as well in the pubertal growth spurt and in maintaining the adult body. However, no one has ever shown any harmful effects of lowering androgen levels in women. The side effects of anti-androgen are generally unrelated to their blocking the effects of androgens on a woman's body.

Although I have discussed some of the androgen antagonists in the stories of my patients, here is specific information on each of the androgen antagonists available in the United States and an important one available only in other countries.

Not all of these drugs were designed to be androgen antagonists. The one most widely used in the United States, spironolactone, was introduced more than thirty years ago as a diuretic and anti-hypertensive. It has these effects because it blocks the salt-retaining hormone aldosterone. Since this hormone is chemically a steroid like the androgens, it is not surprising that spironolactone can block the androgen receptor, just as it can block the aldosterone receptor. While the official labeling of spironolactone does not include androgenic disorders as an indication, it has been very widely used for these conditions;

there are many articles in medical journals confirming its effectiveness.

Most of the other drugs were developed to be androgen antagonists, but they also are not officially labeled for use in hirsutism or other androgenic disorders. In the case of flutamide, extensive studies have been done in Canada demonstrating that it is effective. However, the manufacturer is not planning to do the extensive studies necessary to get FDA approval for an indication for hirsutism in the labeling.

The reasons no manufacturer wants to seek FDA approval for treatment of androgenic disorders with these drugs are economic and political. The process of obtaining FDA approval for a drug indication costs tens of millions of dollars or more and takes several years. Because of worry about birth defects, the FDA is particularly stringent on drugs for benign conditions that will be taken by women of childbearing age. The pharmaceutical companies are also worried about the risk of being sued. This de facto policy of restricting testing of new drugs for menstrual age women aims at protecting them and their unborn children. But it also discriminates against women in this age group because they are denied the benefits of many safe drugs. Fortunately this has now been recognized by the FDA, and manufacturers are now required to include women in their studies of new drugs.

ANTI-ANDROGENS AND PREGNANCY: A WARNING

In general, androgen antagonists are *not* safe during pregnancy because they might interfere with the formation of the genitalia of a male fetus. You should not take an anti-androgen unless you are using an entirely reliable form of contraception. This is especially true of flutamide and finasteride (both discussed later). Theoretically it should be true also of spironolactone, but so far as I know no birth defects have been reported that are attributable to the use of it in pregnancy. I suspect many pregnant women have taken it, especially since it was introduced in the pre-thalidomide era when there was little caution about the use of medication during pregnancy. Nonetheless, if you take spironolactone you must be meticulous about contraception. Even if it turns out not to affect your baby, you do not want to spend your pregnancy worrying.

Anti-androgens and pregnancy do not mix. If you are interested in becoming pregnant within six to twelve months, it is best to delay treatment of your androgenic disorder. Having a child usually has a higher priority than getting rid of androgenic symptoms, although some women are so bothered by unwanted hair, acne, or alopecia that they elect to defer childbearing for a year or two in order to have time for treatment of the androgenic disorder. This kind of decision is highly individual.

For most women, deferring conception for a year or two is not a problem. The old-fashioned idea that complications are unacceptably high after age thirty-five has been revised. However the incidence of Down's syndrome and other genetic abnormalities does increase with the mother's age. If you have actual polycystic ovaries with infrequent periods, there is a strong possibility that you will need hormonal treatment to be able to ovulate and become pregnant. This may be less likely to be successful if you wait because the changes in the ovaries tend to increase over time. Adrenal androgenic disorders, what I have called exaggerated adrenarche, are unlikely to affect fertility. If you have concerns about fertility, the best thing to do is consult a physician who specializes in infertility.

SPIRONOLACTONE

This is the most widely used anti-androgen in the United States; it was introduced more than thirty years ago to block the hormone aldosterone, which raises blood pressure, but it also blocks testosterone and other androgens. Spironolactone also lowers androgen production in some women.

The usual starting dose of spironolactone is 100 mg daily, either as a single dose or divided into two. The latter may work better but is less convenient. The maximum dose is 200 mg per day. Higher doses are used in certain unusual conditions, but I do not recommend them for androgenic disorders. In my experience, 75 mg daily is only occasionally effective, and less is almost never effective. I sometimes see women who have been placed on doses of 50 or even 25 mg a day. After seeing no improvement on these ineffective doses, they understandably become discouraged about spironolactone. Be sure you have been on an adequate dose before giving up on the drug.

It takes a long time for all anti-androgens to work. When acne or seborrhea (excessive oiliness of the skin) is a problem, improvement can be seen within a few weeks because acne is quickly reversible. With hirsutism, seeing a change takes longer. Hair grows in more slowly after three or four months and begins to get lighter and finer during the second six months of treatment. For alopecia, shedding usually slows down and the hair is livelier within a few weeks, but regrowth, if it is to occur at all, may not show itself until the second year of treatment. The reason these changes take so long to appear is the biological nature of hair, which is to grow and change slowly. Other anti-androgens do not seem to work any faster.

Spironolactone is almost always effective to some degree, but some women do not get as much improvement as they would like or deserve. Sometimes it is a matter of continuing the drug longer; in other cases, a different one needs to be tried. If spironolactone has not helped, flutamide (see below) is the next drug to think about. It seems to be a bit more effective, but it is much more expensive and may not be as safe.

Side effects with spironolactone tend to be inconvenient or uncomfortable rather than dangerous or painful. Most common are side effects due to its diuretic action. Only a few women notice having to urinate more often. If you have this problem, try taking the entire dose in the morning so that this effect will be mostly worn off by bedtime. More common than bothersome urinary frequency is very slight dehydration. The symptoms are lightheadedness, especially on standing up quickly, and fatigue. The answer is a simple one: Be sure you drink enough water. Six to eight glasses of eight ounces is the usual recommendation. You can substitute other fluids for plain water, but be careful; many drinks, such as colas or iced tea, contain either sugar or caffeine or both. Common sense and reading labels should allow you to select fluids that are palatable and healthy.

A few women cannot tolerate the diuretic effects of spironolactone because they have too much dizziness. If you spend a lot of time outside in a hot climate and are physically very active, it may be hard for you to drink enough water to keep up with the combined losses from sweat and the diuretic effect. One of my patients worked as a lifeguard in Florida during the summer. The need to be out in the sun and be physically at her strongest in case of the need to rescue someone meant that spironolactone was a problem for her. For most women, however, just being aware of the need to drink enough water usually prevents any problems.

Less common but more annoying is the tendency for spironolactone to make menstrual periods come too close together. It is very common for the interval from one period to the next to be shortened from 28 to 25 or even 22 days. This is usually tolerable, but sometimes periods come as close together as every two weeks. An interval of 21 days or shorter is too frequent. Often this effect of spironolactone is temporary; as the body becomes more used to the drug, menstrual cycles return to a more normal length. If too-frequent periods persist longer than four to six months, however, a way to keep the cycle regulated needs to be found. Lowering the dose returns cycles to normal, but reduces the effectiveness of treatment. Going on birth control pills almost always works, and monthly MPA (medroxyprogesterone acetate; Provera®) sometimes works. The cause of this menstrual change with spironolactone is unknown.

Generic spironolactone tablets are available, but I do not recommend you use generics unless you *absolutely* cannot afford the brand-name product, which is Aldactone® (Searle). Spironolactone is not easily absorbed, and it is critical that the tablet be manufactured properly. Considering that it may take several months before you can tell how well it is working, it does not make sense to take a chance on using a generic. Depending on the dose, Aldactone® usually costs about $50 to $70 per month.

CIMETIDINE

Better known under its brand name of Tagamet®, this was once one of the most widely prescribed drugs in America. As you may know, cimetidine blocks release of acid in the stomach and so helps heal ulcers and milder forms of stomach irritation. More recently other drugs, such as ranitidine (Zantac®, Glaxo), have become more popular for the same purpose. Cimetidine, uniquely in its class of drugs (H2 receptor antagonists), also has some blocking effect on androgen receptors. This may even account for some infrequent side effects, such as gynecomastia (breast development in males.) Spironolactone may occasionally have this effect also though it must be said that most men who take either drug have no problems with them.

Some early studies suggested that cimetidine might help hirsutism, but a more recent one found no effect. My own experience has been like that of this later study; it does not seem to have much effect, even at high doses.

FLUTAMIDE

This drug is newer than spironolactone or cimetidine, having been available in the United States for about four years at the time of this writing. The trade name for flutamide is Eulexin® (Schering-Plough). It was developed specifically as an anti-androgen. Extensive studies show it to be effective for hirsutism, but the labeled indication is for prostatic cancer. (Prostate cells grow in response to androgens, just as breast cells grow in response to estrogen.) Most anti-androgens being introduced now in the United States have prostate disease as their official indication.

In my experience, flutamide is the most effective anti-androgen now available. It has a low incidence of side effects, which are mainly gastro-intestinal upset or diarrhea. Very few women who take flutamide have these problems. There also may be effects on liver enzymes and occasional muscle problems; if you have muscle aches on flutamide, be sure to inform your physician.

Recently there have been reports of severe liver disorders in people receiving flutamide. One was a young adult woman; the rest were older men with prostate cancer. It has not been known to occur in children and the risk to healthy women seems very low—but not zero. For this reason flutamide, despite its effectiveness, should be used only in special situations.

Signs of liver problems from flutamide are jaundice (yellow color of the eyes and skin), tiredness, itching, dark brown urine, light stools, and feeling sick. If these occur flutamide should be stopped at once and your doctor called immediately. The cause of this adverse effect of flutamide is unknown. Fortunately, the liver abnormalities seem to be reversible if the drug is stopped soon enough.

The other drawbacks to flutamide are two: It is very expensive and there is reason to be concerned that it can interfere with development of a male fetus. If you take flutamide, you must use some very reliable method of contraception, such as birth control pills, and be sure to review your contraceptive practices with your doctor.

Cost as well as safety is often a limiting factor in whether a woman can use flutamide, because one month's supply costs about $250. Unfortunately many women who might benefit from flutamide cannot take it for this reason. While it does seem to be moderately more effective than spironolactone and to have fewer side effects—it does not affect the menstrual cycle and has no diuretic effect—these advantages are probably not worth an investment of $3,000 per year for most women. A deciding factor may be what sort of coverage your health insurance gives for medications.

At this time, flutamide has a limited place in the treatment of androgenic disorders, but for some women no other treatment is workable. Other anti-androgens are being developed for treatment of prostate conditions and it is possible some will be useful for androgenic disorders.

KETOCONAZOLE

Like spironolactone and cimetidine, ketoconazole (Nizoral®) was not introduced as an anti-androgen. It is primarily an anti-fungal antibiotic that was later found to be an androgen antagonist. Ketoconazole is effective for androgenic disorders but has one important limitation: It can cause very serious liver injury. If you had a life-threatening fungal infection, you might need to take the chance. But for an androgenic disorder ketoconazole usually is not a good choice.

Ketoconazole comes in topical forms as cream or shampoo. These are safer than the oral forms and may be helpful for seborrheic dermatitis, which is irritation of the skin from excessive oiliness. The cream does not seem to be very effective for acne or hirsutism, probably because the drug does not penetrate deeply enough into the skin.

CYPROTERONE ACETATE

Worldwide, CPA (Androcur®) is the drug most often used for hirsutism. It has been available in Europe for more than twenty years without serious problems. However, the manufacturer has decided not to introduce it here for hirsutism but instead as a treatment for prostatic cancer. This means that the drug will be available in the United States sometime in the future. Safety in pregnancy is not an issue for this drug because it also acts as a contraceptive. Biochemically it is like a super-strong birth control pill or medroxyprogesterone acetate (MPA). Its side effects are like those of MPA. Some women feel fine on it, but a significant number feel bloated or depressed.

I have treated several women with CPA who came to see me from foreign countries where it is available. They have come for return visits or kept me informed of their progress by correspondence. They have had excellent results.

CPA is used in two kinds of regimen. Most common is as the progestin in a special birth control pill called Diane® (Berlex), which contains 2 mg of CPA, and another called Dianette, which is a low-dose pill. These are available in Canada as well as Europe. Some women go there to get it, as current law allows travelers to bring back a limited supply of medicine for their own use, even if it is not FDA-approved in this country.

The other regimens use 25 or 50 mg of CPA for 11 days each month. It is combined with an oral estrogen, which is taken for the first 21 days of the month. This is called the "reverse sequential" or Hammerstein regimen. Because CPA stays in body fat, it needs only to be taken for the first half of the month, but effects persist for the whole month. CPA works well. The problem is that the progestin side effects are very uncomfortable for many women. However, since we now have other anti-androgens available that have fewer side effects, CPA is no longer the best choice for most women.

FINASTERIDE

This drug has recently been introduced by Merck under the trade name Proscar®, as a treatment for prostate disease. Finasteride is not for prostate cancer but the much more common benign prostatic hypertrophy (enlargement of the prostate), which affects a majority of men as they get older. Because the prostate encircles the urethra, when it gets larger the urethra is squeezed and difficulty in passing urine results. The enlargement of the prostate is an effect not of testosterone itself but of dihydrotestosterone (DHT). Hair thinning also seems to be an effect of DHT, rather than of testosterone itself. Since finasteride prevents DHT from being made from testosterone, there is reason to think it might help hirsutism and alopecia. Studies so far are limited, however. It is possible that a topical form will be developed for androgenic disorders.

Finasteride is moderate in cost, about $50 per month. The same cautions about birth defects in male children exposed *in utero* that I discussed with flutamide apply as much or more to finasteride.

TOPICAL ANTI-ANDROGENS

Several pharmaceutical companies are considering developing anti-androgens in skin-cream form. The idea is a good one: to block androgens in the skin, where they cause most of their problems. The question is whether the medication will get deeply enough into the skin to reach the pilosebaceous units. Topical anti-androgens may work, but probably not nearly as well as the oral ones do. They may be useful for men who are concerned about thinning hair. (If men take anti-androgens by mouth, they will have a loss of sex drive and of the ability to have erections.) Topical anti-androgens may be more important for men than women. It will be many years before drugs of this type become available. The only topical androgen now available is ketoconazole (Nizoral®), discussed above.

Lowering Androgens Coming from the Adrenal

Many women with androgenic disorders have what I earlier termed exaggerated adrenarche, or very mild overproduction of androgens by their adrenal glands. A few have much greater overproduction due to adrenal hyperplasia. The treatment for both of these situations is small doses of glucocorticoids to partially suppress the adrenal.

First, remember that what I am saying applies only to overproduction of androgens by the adrenal gland. If the adrenal gland makes too much of its other hormones (cortisol or aldosterone), the situation is much more serious. Because these are not specifically female hormone problems and are rare, I will not cover them in this book.

The best form of glucocorticoid for androgenic disorders is dexamethasone (Decadron®). Prednisone is also used, but because it is shorter-acting I do not think it is as good a choice. If you are considering taking either of these glucocorticoids for an androgenic disorder, you should make yourself sure of two things: that the dose is not too high, and that there is a possibility that it can help you.

Both drugs have been overprescribed for androgenic disorders in the past. They can be helpful, but only if you have increased androgens coming from your adrenal gland. If the problem is in your ovary or simply sensitivity of your pilosebaceous units, dexamethasone or prednisone will not help. There is one exception: brief periods of treatment for infertility. Even with ovarian androgen excess, glucocorticoids will sometimes suppress levels of androgens within the ovary and can help restore ovulation.

For long-term use of dexamethasone, the maximum dose is 0.375 mg daily, but you should start at a dose of 0.125 mg, and increase only if blood tests show that your androgen levels are still high. There is less data about the right doses of prednisone for androgenic disorders, which is one of the reasons I do not use it. However, any dose in excess of 5 mg daily is too much for long-term treatment of these conditions.

It is not necessary or good for you to have your androgens suppressed to zero. To do so requires taking too much dexamethasone. Reasonable levels with suppression are testosterone 40 mg/dl, free testosterone 5 pg/ml, androstenedione 200 ng/dl, and DHEA-S 200 mcg/dl. It is not necessary to have your androgen levels brought down lower than these.

By using moderate doses of glucorticoids your adrenal gland will not be fully suppressed and so will be able to do its job of increasing its secretion of cortisol in the face of the stress. The physical stresses that require extra cortisol include repeated vomiting, high fever, or general anesthesia. If you have been on dexamethasone, prednisone, or any other glucocorticoid and these stresses occur, it is prudent to have an extra amount of glucocorticoid, to be sure your body is protected. I have never seen any problem with the small doses of dexamethasone stated above, but you still should make all of your doctors aware that you are on this medication.

The information in this section applies only to use of dexamethasone and prednisone for adrenal suppression in androgenic disorders. If you are taking glucocorticoids for some other reason, do not assume what I have said applies to you; seek other sources of information. I also recommend that you reread the section in Chapter Two on glucocorticoids if you are taking glucocorticoids or are considering taking them for any reason.

Treatment of Ovarian Androgen Excess

For most women who have increased androgens coming from their ovaries, birth control pills are a simple solution. For women in whom this does not work or who cannot safely or comfortably take the pill, other methods are available. I will discuss the different methods in detail so that if you are considering one, you will have the information you need to decide if it is right for you. Only a few women with ovarian androgen excess will need to consider using a Gn-RH analogue; if you are not one of them, you can skip the discussion of this therapy, unless of course you are simply interested or are considering it for a different condition, such as fibroids or endometriosis.

BIRTH CONTROL PILLS

(See also Chapter Twelve.) The pill suppresses the secretion of follicle-stimulating hormone (FSH) and luteinizing hormone (LH) by the pituitary gland. The result is suppression of ovulation and partial suppression of hormone secretion by the ovary. Any decrease in estrogen and progesterone is not noticed because these hormones are in the pill. But androgens decrease also, and so the pill can be useful for women with androgenic disorders. There are two limitations: The suppression is only partial, so for women with very high testosterone levels, the lowering may not be enough. And there is the possibility of the same side effects and contraindications that affect use of the pill for contraception. However, for many women with mild ovarian androgen excess, the pill is a very effective adjunct to an anti-androgen. This combination is probably more effective than an anti-androgen alone if your ovaries are overproducing androgens. There are other important advantages to this kind of combination. The pill prevents the too-frequent periods that can occur with spironolactone, and it protects against the possibility of pregnancy when the mother is on a drug that might cause a birth defect.

The progestin in some birth control pills is slightly androgenic (see Chapter Twelve). If you already have a problem with too much androgen effect on your body, you should use one of the pills that is least androgenic. This means OrthoCyclen®, OrthoTricyclen®, OrthoCept®, Modicon® (all Ortho-Pharmaceuticals) and Desogen® (Organon), Demulen 35® (Searle), or Ovcon 35® (Mead Johnson Laboratories). How you take the pill is not different for an androgenic disorder than it is for contraception.

Gn-RH ANALOGUES

These are a fascinating group of drugs to endocrinologists because their way of working is extremely subtle. This was discussed in Chapter Three. When treatment with a Gn-RH analogue is started, at first the pituitary gland is stimulated and estrogen levels go up. After a week or a little longer, the pituitary starts to show inhibition. Because the pituitary gland no longer stimulates the ovary, estrogen and ovarian androgen secretion stops. At this point, many women have what seems like a period because, with the fall in estrogen, the endometrium sheds. If Gn-RH analogue therapy is continued (as it usually is, depending on the situation), estrogen levels continue to fall, and the symptoms of estrogen deficiency appear after a few weeks, including hot flashes and vaginal dryness. If the Gn-RH analogue is being used to lower estrogen levels, as is done for fibroids or endometriosis, not much can be done for these estrogen-deficiency symptoms. These usually limit how long therapy can be given, since other estrogen-deficiency problems also begin, especially calcium loss from the bones. But if the purpose is only to lower androgens, estrogen replacement therapy can be given, just as it would be for estrogen deficiency from any other cause.

With this kind of treatment, all the ovarian hormones are suppressed for the sake of lowering androgens. Then the estrogen and progesterone are added back. This may sound complicated and cumbersome, and it is. The ovary is suppressed much more completely than it is with birth control pills, but using a Gn-RH analogue is a lot harder than taking birth control pills. Safety does not seem to be a problem; the Gn-RH analogues appear to have no effects on the body other than lowering FSH and LH. Treatment is expensive; the cost ranges from $200 to $400 per month. If you need an expensive drug, do not give up hope if you can't afford it; check into your insurance situation. Some provide coverage for long-term medication—you may have this benefit and not know about it. Your doctor should be able to give you some help here by writing to your insurance company to explain why the medication is medically necessary.

Gn-RH analogues are destroyed in the stomach if taken orally. This means that they must be taken as a nose spray or by injection. For the most widely used preparation, leuprolide (Lupron®), a depot form is available that lasts for an entire month after it is injected. The nose spray naferelin (Synarel®,

Syntex) needs to be used three times a day, so for most busy women the discomfort of a monthly injection is easier than the bother of using the spray. But the spray does work and is fine, if you prefer it to injections. For some women with severe ovarian androgen excess, using a Gn-RH analogue may be worth the inconvenience. Most women with PCO do not have testosterone levels so high that they need to consider this kind of treatment. For those who do, however, Gn-RH analogues succeed where all other medical treatments fail. Of course, removing the ovaries does the same thing, but it requires surgery and is irreversible.

SURGERY FOR OVARIAN ANDROGEN EXCESS

The problem of ovarian androgen excess was discovered long before the hormones themselves were identified. Because it was noticed that there was an excess of the cells in the interior of polycystic ovaries, the idea was conceived to try to remove some of the extra cells by surgery. A deep wedge of tissue was removed from each ovary, and in many women ovulation was restored and sometimes hirsutism improved somewhat. This operation, called bilateral ovarian wedge resection, was the only treatment available until the 1960s. It is sometimes used today, but rarely in the United States.

I do not recommend this procedure for three reasons. First, it is an operation with general anesthesia and has risks, although they are extremely low for a healthy woman. Second, adhesions in the pelvis may result and impair fertility. Finally and most importantly, the improvement is temporary. Modern hormonal treatment gives much better results. If your concern is to be able to ovulate, then use of FSH and LH or related hormones to induce ovulation is more likely to be successful. If you have extremely high androgen levels but are not concerned about being able to conceive, then it is better to have the entire ovary removed, as wedge resection will not fully or permanently correct the androgen excess. A Gn-RH analogue is a medical alternative to surgery.

Occasionally ovarian androgen excess is due to a tumor. Such a condition requires prompt surgery by a gynecologist specializing in oncology.

Non-hormonal Acne Medications

Without the stimulation of oil production by androgens, there would be no acne; it is at root an endocrine disorder. However, other factors contribute to acne, and many treatments have been devised that work in the later steps of the acne process. Conventional acne treatments all work at these later stages. While they are less effective than hormonal therapy, especially by themselves, they can help acne.

Treatments aimed at skin-surface stickiness and bacterial growth can benefit acne, but because they do not address the cause, they are usually palliative rather than curative. For mild acne, however, they may be all that is necessary. For more severe acne, they may be added to hormonal therapy to speed healing or improve an incomplete response. By themselves, they rarely clear bad acne completely. Unfortunately these are the only treatments offered to most women with acne, because most doctors have been trained to think of acne as a skin disease rather than a hormonal disorder.

If you have mild acne, it is entirely reasonable to try these simple treatments first, especially if you have no other signs of an androgenic disorder such as increased facial and body hair, scalp hair loss, or irregular periods. However, if they do not clear your skin after a few months (assuming you remember to take the pills and apply the topical faithfully), then it is time to seek hormonal evaluation.

If you are already on non-hormonal acne treatment, it is

usually a good idea to continue it until your skin has been cleared by the anti-androgens and other hormonal medications. If you have bad acne and have had no treatment at all, it is reasonable to go right to hormonal treatment, but antibiotics and topicals may be started at the same time for quicker healing. It takes more medicine to clear acne than to maintain the skin in its clear condition. When your skin has been the way you want it for six to twelve months, that is the time to work out a schedule for decreasing the medication.

Let's look at the conventional non-hormonal acne treatments.

ANTIBIOTICS

These have been a mainstay of conventional treatment for decades. They act on the infectious component of acne and inhibit the growth of bacteria that make the sebum more irritating. The most commonly used ones are tetracycline, erythromycin, minocycline (Minocin®, Lederle) and trimethoprim-sulfa (Bactrim®, Roche, or Septra®, Burroughs Wellcome). Of these, minocycline works best, but it is extremely expensive, costing more than $1.50 per capsule. If cost is not a problem for you or the infectious component of your acne is major, as in hidradenitis suppuritiva, for example, then it is the best choice. Tetracycline is similar, is only slightly less effective, and costs only pennies a day. The problem with tetracycline is side effects; photosensitivity (increased susceptibility to sunburn) and vaginal yeast infections occur commonly. If you do not have these problems with tetracycline, it is probably a good medication for you. If you do not know how your body will react to tetracycline, I recommend erythromycin as a better choice. The high doses used for strep throats and other respiratory infections often cause stomach upset or abdominal pain, but the lower dose effective for acne rarely causes these. The dose is usually 250 mg of erythromycin itself or 333 mg of the delayed-release form (E-Mycin®, Boots), both twice a day. The delayed-release form is slightly more expensive but seems to work out better. Because it is less likely to have side effects than tetracycline and is far less expensive than minocycline, erythromycin is the best choice for most women with acne. *One caution: If you are taking one of the new antihistamines, such as terfenacline (Seldane®, Marion Merrill Dow) or astemizole (Hismanol®, Janssen), erythromycin can cause a dangerous drug interaction. Never take these in combination.*

There have been warnings that antibiotics can interfere with the effectiveness of birth control pills, but this is unlikely with the low antibiotic doses used for acne. However, if you are on antibiotics, be extra sure not to forget any of your pills.

Topical antibiotic preparations for acne are helpful and include some containing clindamycin (which is dangerous orally) (Cleocin T® [Upjohn]) and erythromycin (EryGel® Allergan Herbert) or Erycelle® (Ortho Pharmaceutical). Another antibacterial that probably works just as well for most women is benzoyl peroxide, which comes in 5 percent and 10 percent strengths. It is sold over the counter under numerous brand names. The well-known Oxy 5® and Oxy 10® (SmithKline Beecham) are good because they have a non-sticky vehicle that will not clog up your pores further. Benzoyl peroxide preparations must be used every day to work, but many people find their face gets red and irritated from them. There is a simple solution to this: You can use the stronger 10 percent strength after cleaning your face in the evening, but wash it off completely after 30 minutes. If this does not give enough improvement after two or three weeks, you can gradually work up to leaving it on longer. Usually fair skin is more sensitive to the irritation.

RETINOIDS

These are forms of vitamin A that dry the skin and make it less oily. Side effects, as you might expect, are dryness and soreness of the skin. Tretinoin (Retin-A®) is the topical form and has been in use for about twenty years. Hailed as the complete solution to acne when it came out, it has not quite lived up to that promise. The same is true of isotretinoin (Accutane®), an oral vitamin A analogue. Accutane® is more effective, but because the entire body is affected by it there is drying of all skin and mucous membranes. It also can cause changes in the liver. But the most serious problem with Accutane® is that it causes severe birth defects in almost half the fetuses exposed to it in utero, so that Roche devotes most of its marketing efforts to teaching doctors how to educate women on Accutane® to avoid getting pregnant.

For a very few women Accutane® may be necessary, but it must be used very carefully. My experience clearly shows that hormonal therapy, as described in this chapter, gives a better result—the skin simply looks better—without the skin drying and other side effects.

If Accutane® has been recommended to you, I would recommend that you investigate the availability of hormonal treatment first. If you do take it, I suggest a lower dose than usually recommended. Generally 20 mg to 40 mg daily is enough. Treatment is given only for a few months. Be sure your doctor is experienced with it; dermatologists generally are. *A foolproof method of contraception is a must for women on Accutane®.*

For most women, Retin-A® is a better alternative, but it also can cause drying and soreness of the face. I recommend using the 0.025% gel (which is more effective than the cream) and washing it off after 30 minutes. If necessary, you can work up to leaving it on longer, as described for benzoyl peroxide. If your skin is irritated or dry even with this method, try using Retin-A® cream instead.

A few years ago, a study showed that tretinoin might be effective in diminishing wrinkles. So many women had it prescribed for this purpose that for a while there was a shortage; many of my acne patients were unable to find any in drugstores. I would not recommend tretinoin for wrinkles at this time, because its long-term effects in this situation are not certain.

COSMETICS

Acne and oily skin are very common, and the number of personal care products made for them are truly overwhelming. I can only make some suggestions; you may find other things that are as good or better than what I suggest here.

First of all, avoid products that are comedogenic (tending to plug up the pores and cause pimples). Worst are those with petroleum jelly or other mineral oils. These can make acne worse. Old-fashioned cold creams also tend to be comedogenic. Cosmetic lines that are designed for the needs of women with skin problems include Almay, Clinique, and Prescriptives. Chanel also makes certain products designed for oily skin, including a special moisturizer called Base Pureté. Many physicians tell their patients that more expensive brands like these are no better than cheaper ones sold in drugstores. I am unconvinced. Even allowing for the fact that much of the cost of these goes for packaging, the quality of the ingredients is still better. On the other hand, high cost does not guarantee a good product. Some trial and error is necessary on the part of the user. Almay tends to be lower-priced than the other brands I have mentioned.

There are special concerns for black women. Cosmetics and hair dressings often contain petroleum jelly or similar substances. These usually exacerbate acne. Products that are oil-free are better.

There are many special skin cleansers. Astringents contain

alcohol and dry the skin. They have a slight sting, which makes it feel as if your skin is cleaner. However, they add little to the effects of a good soap and can cause irritation or dryness. The Clinique face soaps are excellent and last a long time. For women with acne, the soap for oily skin is usually the best. A variety of mild abrasive scrubs are sold by Clinique and other cosmetic companies. These are somewhat controversial. They do help remove the dead skin cells, but they can irritate and slightly injure the skin if you use them too often (more than once every one to two days) or push very hard while scrubbing in eagerness to help get rid of acne. These cleansers are not necessary if you wash your face twice a day with soap. On the other hand, if you like the effect, by all means use one, but rub it over your skin very gently. Mud masks remove oil temporarily, but do not do anything for acne. My recommendation is to use these sort of special cleaning products only if you like them, but to save your money to buy the best quality soap.

Opaque foundations are the best way to cover acne. More "sheer" makeup will not cover as effectively. Heavy cover-up foundation may conceal the unevenness of pigmentation that results from long-standing acne but may accentuate the pitting. In using blush, remember that darkening something will make it seem to recede, and lightening it will make it seem to come forward. Therefore pits should be lightened and bumps darkened.

When your acne is successfully treated, you may find yourself with a skin problem you never imagined could happen to you: dryness. Retin-A® and Accutane® are drying. Anti-androgenic therapy is not drying in itself, but it does take away the excessive oiliness that may have kept your skin from drying out in the winter. You simply need to start doing what most women have to do in northern climates in the winter: Use moisturizer. Here again choosing the proper product is important, and oily ones should be avoided. In my opinion, one of the very best, which is manufactured by a dermatologist, is MI FINE Skin lotion (Michel Skin Care Enterprises, Cleveland, Ohio 44122); it is not widely distributed but can be ordered by telephone (1-800-331-SKIN). Other good series of moisturizer products are Nivea and Vaseline Intensive Care.

ACNE AND FOOD

Acne is not the result of diet. Specifically, greasy cheeseburgers, milk shakes, chocolate, and french fries do not cause acne. This superstition about foods causing acne is not unique to Americans; the Chinese believe acne to result from eating foods that cause too much "internal hot air." Fried foods are included in this group, but so are spicy foods like chili and curry, along with alcoholic drinks. Although there are good reasons for avoiding greasy foods, acne is not one of them. I suspect this ubiquitous belief is simply due to the fact that skin with acne looks greasy and that teenagers tend to eat a lot of greasy foods. Changing your diet to a low fat one is certainly good for you, but it will not cure your acne.

Life with an Androgenic Disorder

I think most women who develop an androgenic disorder feel that their life is not quite the same as a result. There is the need for extra time with grooming and makeup. Even with good relationships and friends, there is always a certain insecurity that the problem will be detected and held against you. And there is the fear the problems will get worse. Finally, there are medicines to be taken and doctors to be visited. Treatments for androgenic disorders are very good and have made a major difference in the lives of many women, but it is still not the same as if you'd never had the problem.

Unwanted Hair Removal

For the women I see as patients, local removal has not worked. There is too much hair to remove or, because of the hair's darkness and thickness, stubble remains visible. Doctors sometimes have the misconception that removing or bleaching hair is all women ever need as a means of dealing with the problem. As anyone with hirsutism knows, this is far from the case. However, local hair removal does have a place in self-care for most women with increased hair growth. It does not substitute for hormonal treatment, but rather supplements it. For women with only a few unwanted hairs, local removal will be enough, but I suspect that if you have read this far in this chapter, you are not in this group. Women who remove hair, whether a lot or a little, do need advice on how to do it.

PLUCKING

This is the most commonly used method, employed especially on the chin. The chin is the area of the face that is most sensitive to androgens, and most women have at least an occasional unwanted hair on it. Many women use tweezers to pluck a few chin hairs each morning before putting on their makeup. This is not really a good method because pulling the hair out by the root injures the skin, causing inflammation and sometimes infection. Over a long period of time, the chronic inflammation gives an irregular, almost lumpy, appearance to the skin of the chin. As new hairs grow in, they may become ingrown, producing a pimple-like infection. Nonetheless, I have to admit that few women I talk to are willing to give up plucking, because nothing else is quite so easy and effective. And for the woman who needs to remove one or two hairs every few days, plucking is perfectly satisfactory because scarring is unlikely. But if you are spending a significant amount of time every morning pulling out hairs, I would recommend that you find a better method.

WAXING

This is less common than plucking, but the principle is the same: pulling the hair out from the root. Wax is put on an area of skin, allowed to dry completely and then pulled off. Waxing is usually done in beauty parlors or spas, you really cannot do it yourself. This is one of its disadvantages: Waxing is relatively expensive. It also can injure the skin.

Of all methods of hair removal, waxing produces the best short-term aesthetic result. The skin looks entirely free of hair and is smooth to the touch. The hair does grow back eventually, but this usually takes two or three weeks, because the hair has been removed all the way down to the root rather than at the surface of the skin. However, for the woman whose hormones are causing her to have rapid body hair growth, waxing does not last as long, and doing it every few days is impractical, as well as painful and traumatic to the skin. Waxing works best for the woman who wants hair removed from a large area of skin for a limited duration, for example, before a vacation on the beach. It is not suitable for long-term control of hirsutism.

DEPILATORIES

Depilatories are creams containing chemicals that dissolve the hair. They are left on a very short time—usually one to four minutes—then thoroughly removed. The problem with depilatories is that the proteins on the surface of the skin are quite similar to those that hair is made of. If left on even slightly too long, depilatories will start to dissolve keratin, the surface protein of the skin. The result is a burn, with the skin becoming temporarily painful and reddened. Serious injuries are unlikely, but many women stop using depilatories because their skin is raw afterward. It is critical that you time carefully how long the depilatory remains on your skin; you should be watching the clock the whole time from when you put it on to when it is time to wash it off, so it will not remain on any extra seconds. Finding the right length of time to leave on a depilatory is tricky. If left on too long they burn, but if removed too soon they do not fully dissolve the hair. This is mainly a problem with facial hair; the skin of the legs, thighs, and abdomen is far less delicate than that of the face, and there seem to be fewer problems with irritation at these locations.

If you remove facial hair, it is worth trying a depilatory because it is less injurious to the skin than plucking or waxing. Be sure the one you pick is designed for use on the face. Time it carefully. Begin with the shortest application time recommended in the instructions contained in the package. If the hair was not fully removed but your skin was not irritated, you can leave it on fifteen to thirty seconds longer the next time you try it, which should not be sooner than twenty-four hours. Using it repeatedly on the same day is certain to be very irritating to your skin. If you get a good result in terms of hair removal but have some irritation, a useful treatment is to apply 1% hydrocortisone cream to the skin right after washing off the depilatory, after drying your face completely. The hydrocortisone has a very mild anti-inflammatory effect, and use every few days will not harm your skin.

I have not found many women who are enthusiastic about use of depilatory, but it does work well for some. It is certainly worth trying and experimenting with the application time to see if you can get it to work out for you.

RAZORS

Although it is understandably not very popular among women, shaving is the best method of removing hair because it is least traumatic to the skin. This is especially true now because of technological advances in the design and manufacture of disposable razors.

Women do not like to use razors on their faces and necks for two reasons. The first is emotional; shaving is regarded as a masculine activity. Second is the fear that shaving will cause the hair to grow in thicker and darker and that shaving will ultimately make the problem worse. Neither idea is entirely true.

The belief that using a razor to remove facial hair will result in it coming in darker and thicker is universal. I have encountered it when lecturing in several foreign countries as well as in the United States. Nonetheless, it is not true. I think there are two reasons for this idea. The first has to do with how a razor works. It cuts off hair at the skin surface, where it is thick. As the hair grows out, the end of the cut hair is thicker than the tapering tip of an uncut hair. Hair growing back after being cut by a razor *feels* thicker, but that is because when you run your hand along your face, you feel the thicker shaft rather than the finer tip of a totally new hair.

There is another reason. Unwanted facial and body hair tends to increase over time. Often a woman will start using a razor when she first notices an increase in hair. Some months or years later, the hair is even thicker, and the use of the razor is blamed. But the increased thickness and darkness would have happened anyway. It was due to the underlying hormone problem that caused her to start using a razor in the first place.

Now I do not expect to convert many women to the use of the razor for removal of facial hair. The major point of this book is to explain hormonal treatments that can usually make such methods unnecessary anyway. But I do want to reassure those women who use a razor because it is the only thing that works for them. Shaving is a good method for hair removal, and you are not in any way harming yourself or making the hair growth worse if you use it. If you have been afraid to use a razor but have facial hair you think may be very noticeable, the razor may be part of the solution for you. To get a good result, attention to the details of selecting and using a razor is important.

Women have two special needs with respect to razor use. They want to avoid irritating or injuring their softer skin, and they generally want to cut the hair off as close as possible to the skin so that no hair will show. The great advantages of razors are that they are specifically designed to remove facial hair and that they minimize injury to the skin. A limitation of razors is that their edge is straight, but the skin of the face is not. This is not so great a problem on the leg because the soft tissue underneath the skin can adapt to the flat edge of the razor.

One disposable razor, the Gillette Sensor®, is a good choice. It has twin blades, which cut better and with less irritation. Also the blades are floated on springs so that they follow the contours of the skin. Because the Sensor® blades follow the organic contours of the skin, they remove hair more effectively and are less irritating. Sensor comes in a woman's version. The blades are the same as the razor marketed for men, but there is a strip with special moisturizers and aloe, which make it kinder to a woman's more tender skin. The handle is wider, making it more comfortable for women to use.

For women who use a razor for hair removal, proper skin preparation should be as much a part of regular skin care as cleansing and moisturizing. The most important first step is to wet the hair for at least three minutes. This allows the hair shaft to take up water. This is easy when shaving the legs, since most women do it in the bathtub or shower. But it takes a special effort to thoroughly soak the hairs on the face.

The next step is to apply a shaving cream or gel. As with razor blades, shaving cream technology has also improved. Lubricants and moisturizers result in less scraping of the skin and therefore less soreness. So far as I know, there are no shaving skin preps designed specifically for women, but certain of those whose marketing is aimed toward men are especially suitable for women. Gels are better than creams but are less popular because they do not feel as good when being put on. Edge Gel® is excellent and has the advantage of coming in an unscented version. The Gillette Series® Gel is also excellent.

Gillette Foamy® and the newer Gillette Series Foam® are both good. Drakkar Noir makes two, of which I prefer the slightly more expensive High Performance Moisture Shave®. Aramis Foam® contains the local anesthetic benzocaine, which reduces the discomfort of shaving. Using soap to wash your face before applying cream or gel will further soften the hairs.

If you still find your skin is irritated, even after use of these products, be sure you are leaving the gel or cream on for about two minutes before using the razor. Most women do not bother with shaving creams or gels, but instead use soap. This seems like less of a bother; however, while it may be enough for the legs, it is not for the more tender skin of the face. After using a razor, be sure to apply a moisturizer once your face is clean and dry afterward, as this will decrease irritation. Even though there may be enough hair to require frequent removal, a woman's skin is delicate and still requires tender care.

ELECTROLYSIS

Electrolysis has been controversial at times. Some women have a good experience with it; others do not. Because it can make a major difference for some women, it is important to understand electrolysis, what it is, what it can do, and what it cannot do.

Electrolysis refers to destruction—"lysis"—of the hair follicle using an electric current. A related method, thermolysis, uses heat. There are a variety of other methods, such as the so-called "electronic tweezers" and a home version called the Epilady®.

Some of these methods work, but many do not. Unfortunately the consumer has no easy way to learn if the method she has chosen, perhaps through an advertisement, is truly effective. Electrolysis is effective only if the probe or needle is put down into the hair follicle. If the current is only applied to the hair itself or to the surface of the skin, it will not permanently remove the hair. The so-called electric tweezers are supposed to transmit electricity down the hair into the follicle but, in fact, hair does not conduct electricity. Methods like this are no better than plucking. Real electrolysis requires a high degree of technical skill. The other techniques are easy ways out; like most such easy ways, they do not work.

There is a certain amount of discomfort in electrolysis because of the electric current. A highly skilled electrologist can minimize this by setting the current properly, but all effective methods involve some pain, although it is slight. It is more uncomfortable for some women than for others. When done under a doctor's supervision, local anaesthetic can be applied to the skin, but this is not completely effective because it does not penetrate deeply enough.

Another problem with electrolysis is that it can leave tiny dark marks at the sites where the needle has been applied. This is because there is a certain amount of inflammation after the hair follicle has been exposed to the current. Inflammation usually results in darkening of the skin of the inflamed area. Women differ in their susceptibility to this condition. Some develop it with any minor injury to their skin; others usually escape visible changes. Dark-complected Caucasian as well as black and Asian women are most likely to show visible darkening simply because they are genetically programmed to have deeper pigmentation everywhere. The dark marks tend to fade over time but may not become completely invisible.

I suggest that if you try electrolysis you have the first few treatments on areas of the face that are not directly visible, such as under the chin. If you do not develop skin darkening where you have had the electrolysis, you can continue the treatments in more exposed areas. But if you notice small dark spots a few weeks after the area was treated, you should continue only if you can accept similar marks where they will be more visible. Most women who try electrolysis find that the discomfort and the pigmentary changes are quite acceptable, but you need to try it out for yourself before committing to long-term treatment.

Electrolysis works hair by hair; so, properly done, it is a slow process. The more hairs you want removed, the longer it will take and the higher will be the cost. An experienced electrologist should be able to give you some estimate of the amount of time required to get the result you want. Usually it will take several months for noticeable progress to be made.

Those women who have a relatively small number of hairs that are highly visible—for example, on the upper lip—get the best result with electrolysis. Others who have less obviously visible hairs, but many more of them, are the ones likely to end up frustrated. It may simply take too long to remove all the unwanted hair. Progress on the cheeks and sideburns tends to be slower than on the upper lip and chin, simply because there are usually so many more hairs on these larger surfaces.

Electrolysis is permanent in the sense that the hair follicle, once treated, will not grow another hair. However, other follicles become active, and this creates the appearance of hairs growing back. Whether electrolysis will be effective in reducing the amount of hair on a particular area of skin will depend on the relative rates of removal and appearance of new hairs. If there is a strong drive to hair growth due to hormones stimulating the hair follicles, it is hard for electrolysis to keep up with it, and there may not seem to be much decrease in hair. However, if a woman has a stable amount of facial hair, the results of electrolysis are often quite satisfying.

If you are considering electrolysis, be sure you select a skilled electrologist. There are two professional organizations whose members generally adhere to high standards: the American Electrolysis Association and the Electrolysis Guild. The former is a large organization; the latter is more selective. Either will provide a referral to a member in your area if you call. I strongly recommend this method rather than using the Yellow Pages or responding to advertisements. There are too many practitioners who are inadequately skilled, and you do not want to find this out after months of ineffective treatment. It is also important that proper equipment be used. The one I am most familiar with is the Instatron, made by the Instatron Corporation in Rhode Island.

There is another matter that you must inform yourself about when you start electrolysis, and that is whether your electrologist uses disposable needles. *Under no circumstances should you have electrolysis performed except with a disposable needle!* This should be more than obvious in this era of awareness of AIDS and other blood-transmitted infections. Yet not all electrologists use them. Sterilization and reuse is fine in theory, but because it requires a degree of technical knowledge of sterilization procedures, which electrologists may not have, it may not always work in practice. Insist on use of a disposable needle.

I do not see hormonal therapy and electrolysis as competing treatments but as complementary. If you have a relatively few unwanted hairs and no sign of a hormonal disorder (such as irregular periods), electrolysis may be enough for you. If you have more extensive hair coverage, however, electrolysis by itself is less likely to get you to where you want to be. If you have had optimal hormonal therapy but have not gotten rid of all the hair that bothered you, electrolysis might be considered to further decrease remaining hair. It is much more efficient to have electrolysis after being on hormonal therapy because there are fewer hairs that need to be treated.

FINAL COMMENTS ON LOCAL HAIR REMOVAL

Considering that half of American women use one or more of these methods, they cannot be all bad. For a few extra hairs, one or more of these methods are all that is needed. There is no need for a trip to the doctor and an extensive endocrine workup if you have only a few hairs at the corner of your upper lip or pluck one or two from your chin every few days. But for women with androgenic disorders, local removal does not give an adequate result. Hormonal therapy can dramatically reduce the amount and thickness and darkness of facial and body hair for most women. If you are troubled by extra hair, whether a lot or a little, there is something that will help.

Androgenic Disorders and Relationships

Whether a woman has facial or body hair or acne seems not to be of particular concern to most men. Nor have I ever known a man to comment on a woman having thin scalp hair. These are just not the things that matter to a man. There are possibly some men who are turned off by extra hair on a woman but there are also some who find it highly erotic. Since this is not a culturally sanctioned preference, men who feel it are unlikely to admit it, while other preferences, notably that for very large breasts, are openly acknowledged. Of the more than one thousand women I have seen with hirsutism, I only know of two or three instances in which their husbands or boyfriends seemed concerned. In these, the real problem in the relationship was something else.

We might also ask, do women notice? Perhaps they do, more than men, but still not very much. My evidence for this is my experience that almost all the women I see because of their concern about hirsutism or alopecia imagine they are the only ones with the problem. Surely those who have it would be able to spot it on other women, yet most never do.

There is one person who will consistently notice any extra hair or other androgenic changes: yourself. You are also the most important person who has to be comfortable with your looks. You have the right to do what you can to look the way you feel you should. Of course you do need to make an informed decision based on a full explanation of any proposed treatments. Not all people, even doctors, realize how important it is for people to be comfortable with their appearance. They think that if your extra hair does not bother them, it should not bother you. Many doctors do understand, but there are others who do not. It is worth calling first to find out if a particular endocrinologist, gynecologist, or dermatologist is interested in working with women who are concerned about androgenic skin or hair problems.

What I have been saying does not mean that I endorse society's emphasis on a woman's appearance. I do not. Unfortunately, our culture is hypocritical about looks and "vanity." We are judged on looks but we're not supposed to care. It is not vain to want to be satisfied with how your body looks, and not something to feel puritanical guilt about. At the same time, accepting that there is a relationship between appearance and self-esteem does not mean you have to regard your appearance as the most important thing in life. But usually the best way to be less concerned with acne, facial hair, or hair loss is to have it properly treated.

Chapter Seven

•

Alopecia:
When Women Start
to Lose Their Hair

$\mathcal{D}$eanna, one of my first patients with alopecia, first came to see me almost ten years ago, referred by her dermatologist. She was twenty-eight, with a curly hair style that gave her an appealingly youthful and lively look. Deanna was cheerful and easy-going, except when it came to what she had come to see me about: her hair loss. In my inexperience at that time, I was not even sure she really had lost any hair; certainly it did not look thin from the top, although Deanna insisted that it had been much fuller a year or two ago. The vertex, the rounded point of the back of the head, did show some thinning, but it was quite mild. Deanna was irritated when something I asked her seemed to suggest that I did not believe she was really losing hair. Like many women with alopecia, she had become sensitized to doctors seeming not to believe she was really losing her hair. When I first started seeing women with alopecia, my colleague endocrinologists were amused and warned me that patients with alopecia were very neurotic. They assumed I would soon realize this and stop seeing women worried about their hair.

Deanna seemed to confirm this impression. As she talked more to me of her life, I learned that she worked as an office manager and enjoyed her career. She had a boyfriend of several years in what sounded like a good relationship. But then she told me that she would not go out of the house except to go to work. She insisted that her boyfriend visit her there. She, of course, did not mind being seen by family members—she lived with her parents—but avoided being in situations with strangers. When she went out, Deanna told me, she thought people were always staring at the back of her head. Going to a movie or concert was especially disturbing to her because the back of her head was visible to many people with nothing else to do as they waited for the show except stare.

Fortunately I had begun to work with Doctor Wilma Bergfeld, the medical pioneer in studying and treating women's hair problems. From her I learned the hormonal basis and fundamentals of treatment for this condition.

When the lab report came back, all Deanna's hormone levels were normal. The androgens were in the lower half of the normal range. This might have led me to adapt my colleagues attitude toward alopecia in that Deanna had no endocrine disease that might be found described in a textbook. Yet something was bothering her, and intuition told me that I should not dismiss it as psychological. Her tests were normal, but there *was* a change in her hair. The pattern would be termed androgenic alopecia had it been worse or had her androgen levels been higher. So it seemed to me reasonable to treat it as if it was androgenic alopecia. I prescribed spironolactone (see Chapter Six), reviewed possible side effects, and suggested she return for a follow-up visit in three more months.

When Deanna came back three months later, she seemed to be no better. She was still distressed enough about her alopecia to avoid going out. She did not think that it was worse, but it was certainly not any better. I did not know then that the first sign of success when treating androgenic alopecia is that shedding slows down. Deanna was having a good initial response. I did tell her that it was too early to tell how well the spironolactone would work and encouraged her to continue with the medication, since she was not having any side effects or problems.

At her next visit nine months later, Deanna still hadn't grown any more hair. She did seem a little less worried, however, because there had been no progression. All along, I had pointed out to Deanna that she actually had a normal amount of hair, that it might be less than she had before but was no less than many other women have. But Deanna was still unhappy about it. I reassured her that there was still a definite chance of her hair returning, that hair changes very slowly, and that it was worth being patient and trying longer. I thought this to be honest advice, but I then had much less certainty about it than I do now, having seen at least 1,000 alopecia patients.

Deanna's next visit was a year and three months after she had started the spironolactone. When I first caught sight of Deanna, I could tell something was different. Her hair was lively and attractive, but then it had never looked bad to me. The problem had been how it had looked to Deanna herself. But what was clearly new was that Deanna was smiling. As I sat down, she told me that her hair was a little fuller. The change was not an enormous one, but she was sure there was improvement. I was relieved that the treatment had worked, that Deanna had not taken medication in vain, and, most of all, that the hair thinning that made her so unhappy was starting to improve. But Deanna admitted she was still unsure about going out of the house; she was happy that there had been some benefit but also afraid that there would not be more. And at this early stage of my experience I could not tell her how much more change there would be. Even now the exact response of alopecia to treatment is sometimes difficult to predict.

Over the next several years, Deanna continued to take the

spironolactone and to come for follow-up visits about every six months. Her hair progressively improved, and her attitude toward herself improved with it. She started going out of the house, enjoying a much fuller social life with her friends and boyfriend. Although she continued to live at home, she no longer led the constricted life she had when I had first seen her. Deanna is now married and happy with her life. Although her hair never grew to be quite as full as it had been before the alopecia started, it improved considerably from what it had been before treatment.

Those who have never had a hair loss problem may not have reflected on how important a full head of hair is to a woman. The purpose of hair is aesthetic, and it's valued all the more because its purpose is to adorn rather than to serve any purely biological purpose. Hair is practically the only part of our body that we can change and adapt to our individuality.

In my experience, there are few physical changes as distressing to a woman as loss of her hair. I am not saying that hair loss is as significant as cancer or heart disease. But if you are the one who has it, alopecia becomes very important and very serious. Mature women, women who have weathered many adversities in their lives, sometimes break down and cry as they talk to me about how distressing their alopecia is and how frustrated they have been in their efforts to get help. This cuts across all divisions among people. I have seen teenage girls, college students, women in their sixties and seventies, Americans, Chinese, Japanese, Indians, Europeans, Middle Easterners, wealthy socialites, women on welfare, scientists, nurses, physicians, single and married women, factory workers, housewives, policewomen, a car mechanic, models, cancer survivors, women with multiple sclerosis, anorexics, the very obese. The misery felt by women who are losing their hair cuts across all possible categories and becomes universal.

I believe the experience of a disease—or a physical change— is just as important as its technical explanation. If you have alopecia, you will want to know why you are having it and you will want to find a treatment. But you also need to know that you are not alone in your feelings. If you are concerned that you may be losing hair, you can at least take modest comfort in knowing that millions of other women have the same problem and are very distressed by it, too. This concern is not "neurotic." It is normal to feel distress at the loss or threatened loss of your hair.

Sherrie was another early patient of mine. At thirty-eight, she was somewhat older than Deanna, but her alopecia had begun at about the same age. Since then, it had gradually progressed so that there was no question that she had thin hair. Sherrie worked as the executive director of a large voluntary organization. Much of her work consisted of fund-raising, as well as giving frequent presentations to varied groups regarding her organization's activities. She was before the public every day. Slender and fashionably but conservatively dressed, Sherrie told me, "I do not think I am much more vain than anyone else, but I know my appearance affects how people receive me and that's what my work is. I really do not know what will happen if I lose much more hair. And I have an active social life which I like and want to keep."

Sherrie had more severe hair loss than Deanna; her scalp was clearly visible when one looked at her head from the top. She used a perm and mousse to give body to her hair, which made her alopecia much less obvious. I reassured her that her hair looked nice—it did—and that I was sure her appearance would help her in her work, not the contrary. Sherrie pointed out that the extra time she needed to spend arranging it in the morning was a problem for her, although one to which she did not see any solution. Sherrie put her concern this way, "When I get up to give a talk at a luncheon, I want to feel the audience is listening to what I say, not staring at my hair." I told her I thought it was very unlikely that anyone thought her hair had anything wrong with it. She agreed that this was

Figure 8.

Alopecia:
Where Women's Hair May Thin

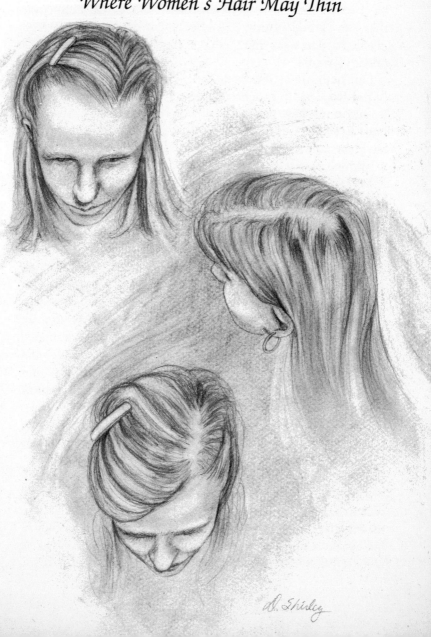

264 THE GOOD NEWS ABOUT WOMEN'S HORMONES

probably so, but added, "I just don't want to be thinking about it. I've always felt confident in public, and I want to continue to. I know my hair is different, and I can't help but worry that others will notice." Sherrie had brought several small plastic bags to show me the hairs she had lost each day of the previous week.

Unlike Deanna, Sherrie did not avoid social contact because of her alopecia. In order to do the kind of work she did, she'd learned long ago to master whatever social insecurities she had. Even had she been unable to get help, Sherrie would have continued to be in the public eye, but her stress level would have gone up considerably.

Sherrie believed my reassurance that most people would not notice her alopecia and that, if they did, it would not affect the way they felt about her. But still she did not feel comfortable with it. "I don't just want to be told to live with it. I want my hair back." Sherrie had some other androgenic changes as well. She'd always had to remove some facial hair, although she found this much less disturbing than the alopecia, as do most women who have both. And her periods had been irregular for many years. She was a little surprised that I showed concern about this and suggested that it needed to be evaluated and treated. "My other doctors told me it didn't matter if I wasn't trying to get pregnant, and I've gotten used to not knowing when my period will come. But you're right. It must not be normal to get your period only a few times a year."

Sherrie's tests showed her testosterone level to be 72 ng/ml, just above the normal range. Her androstenedione and DHEA-S were lower. I explained to her that a testosterone of 72 was high enough to be causing her hair to shed. A dexamethasone suppression test showed that the testosterone was half from her ovaries and half from her adrenals. This meant that suppressing her adrenals with dexamethasone or her ovaries with an oral contraceptive were about equally likely to be effective. Both might need to be used, but only if she did not get a good result with one. It was agreed that she would use an oral contraceptive, since this would also regulate her cycle. Since Sherrie was a non-smoker, her age of thirty-eight was not a problem. Had she smoked, I would not have given her the pill because of the risk of heart disease in women over thirty-five who smoke. I also prescribed spironolactone in the usual starting dose of 50 mg twice a day.

When Sherrie came back for her three-month follow-up visit she was very clear that she had not seen any difference. She'd understood that there would not be any regrowth so soon, but she felt she was still shedding too much. The need to take medicine twice a day was something she found difficult. "I'm usually in my car, then on my way to a dinner or a meeting. It's just too hard and I often forget." She went on, "I really want this to work. Is there something else you can do?"

Scientific rigor would have had me insist to Sherrie that she take the medication for at least six to nine months before increasing the dosage and that she take it twice a day. But she was candid with me that neither was right for her. So we agreed that the spironolactone dose each day would be increased from 100 mg to 200 mg and that she could take it all as a single dose in the morning.

Six months later, Sherrie was guardedly optimistic. "I've been remembering my medicine, and it seems to be working. I'm not shedding so much anymore." It is now two and a half years since Sherrie began treatment. Although her hair looks fuller, she has not had any regrowth (why this happens is explained below). But she has kept what she had. Relieved of the anxiety that she'd end up with practically no hair, Sherrie is much less worried about it. "I feel I can give the energy I spent worrying about my hair to other things," she told me. "When I speak or go to meetings, I do not have to worry that soon I'll be wearing a wig. I'd like to have more come back, but so long as it does not get any thinner than it is now, I can live with it." Fortunately Sherrie came for treatment before

her alopecia had become marked. That it would have continued to worsen I have no doubt, because she'd had steady
loss for nearly a decade and when androgenic alopecia has
progressed steadily like that it usually continues to do so.

Sherrie may still see some regrowth, but it is also possible
that she will not. For this reason, I am pleased that she is
comfortable with the amount of hair she now has and will be
satisfied to be able to hold on to that. For most women with
androgenic alopecia, this is a realistic goal.

There is another benefit to treatment that women receive
even if they do not have actual regrowth. This is that the hair
becomes more vibrant-looking. Endocrine therapy—which
consists of blocking androgens, and when necessary, lowering
their levels—makes women's hair look better. Within a few
weeks of treatment, women with androgenic alopecia usually
have hair that is fuller, livelier, brighter, stronger, and less
likely to break off. All these changes give the appearance of
more hair. One likely factor is that blocking the androgens
decreases the oiliness of the skin and scalp. When the excessive
androgenic activity is corrected with properly selected medication, the skin and hair are no longer too oily and look as they
should.

Judy, another patient of mine, also had alopecia, but with
a different hormonal cause than Sherrie or Deanna. She was
forty-eight, the mother of three children, and, like Sherrie,
socially very active. In earlier years, she'd had no problems
with hair loss, or for that matter anything else related to her
hormones. When she consulted me, her periods were still
monthly and she had no hot flashes, or so it seemed. Once
she thought about it, however, she recalled that she sometimes
felt a little warm although, as she put it, "I'd always been cold-
blooded before." Judy's hair loss had begun about eighteen
months earlier, but the shedding had gotten worse recently.
Although her blonde hair and fair skin made for less contrast

between scalp and hair, so that the alopecia was not conspicuous, a careful look confirmed that her hair was indeed thinning.

Judy's hair loss turned out to be due to the estrogen deficiency of the early stage of menopause. Not all women start to lose hair at menopause, but many do, far more than ever seek treatment for it. The pattern of thinning is practically identical to androgenic alopecia but the cause is different—though still hormonal—and so the treatment is different. (See Chapter Thirteen for discussion of menopausal hair loss and estrogen treatment for it.)

Androgenic Alopecia

Deanna and Sherrie both have androgenic alopecia. Androgenic alopecia is sometimes considered the mild female form of male-pattern baldness. It is true that androgens cause hair to gradually thin in most men and some women. However, the patterns of hair loss are quite different. In men, recession of the front hairline is nearly universal. In women with androgenic alopecia, the anterior hairline is almost always preserved. A few women naturally have a hairline that is back farther than usual, but this simply gives the appearance of a high forehead. Women with androgenic alopecia do not look like bald men. The very different hormonal conditions in a woman's body protect her hair even when the protection does not work perfectly.

Deanna's hair-loss pattern is the most common one in women with androgenic alopecia. Her hair loss was mild, although this was in part due to the fact that she came to me relatively early. The place her hair was thinnest was the vertex, the rounded point at the back of the head. Next most affected was the top or crown of the head. Another place that can be affected is the temples. Although the hairline usually does not recede there, there can be areas of thinning just behind it on the temples. This is usually easy to conceal.

I grade hair loss as mild, moderate, or marked. With mild alopecia there may be a little area of scalp visible at the vertex. (In fact, this is the thinnest area for everyone's hair.) On the crown, there is a slight widening of the space between the hairs where they emerge from the scalp; this is not evident unless the hair is lifted up. Mild alopecia may be very noticeable to the woman who has it, but usually not to others. With moderate alopecia, the scalp is slightly visible from above, and the hair looks thin, but it is still possible to conceal the scalp with styling. When alopecia is marked, the scalp clearly shows through on top. There are intermediate grades as well. Most women I see are in the mild to moderate range. However, many women with minimal or mild alopecia are not aware that their hair is slightly thin. Marked androgenic alopecia is not at all common and usually takes many years to develop. If you are concerned about a lesser degree of alopecia, now is the time to look into treatment so as to prevent it from progressing.

I have talked of hair shedding and thinning as if they were interchangeable, but actually there is a subtle distinction between the two. Thinning is the decrease in hair remaining on the scalp. Shedding is the actual loss of hairs. They sound the same, but they are not because new hair is always growing in to replace that which is shed. The hair that you see or comb is the net of what grows in minus what falls out. If shedding is increased, thinning may occur, but does not always, because more hair may be growing in to replace it. Normally a woman will lose between 100 and 150 hairs every day. Most women do not pay attention to this, even when they are cleaning the drain in the shower, washing their hair, or brushing it off a sweater or dress. It is quite another matter for a woman who has alopecia. Once someone becomes aware of hair loss, seeing all the hairs that have been shed is always alarming.

To judge what is happening with your alopecia, you need to look at what is there in the mirror rather than what is falling out. Focusing on what is shed tends to make the situation look worse than it really is because you cannot see the hairs growing in to take their place. However, changes in shedding are important in judging whether treatment is starting to be effective. The first sign that alopecia is improving is often a slowing of the rate of shedding.

Androgenic alopecia tends to be progressive, although the rate of progression is hard to predict. If progression is rapid, it will probably continue to be so. The same is not necessarily true when progression is slow, since it may become more rapid. This uncertainty is frustrating because it is hard for women with alopecia to know what will happen without treatment. Fortunately most women with androgenic alopecia have only very gradual progression.

Because androgenic alopecia is gradual, it is usually hard to pinpoint when it began. When I did some statistics on my patients a few years ago, I found that, on average, women with androgenic alopecia had the condition about ten years before coming to see me. It was not that they weren't bothered earlier, but that they had trouble finding a doctor who took alopecia seriously and knew how to treat it.

Some hair shedding is temporary, with all growing back within a few months. This kind of unusually heavy shedding has the elegant name of telogen effluvium. The problem is the one I have been describing: It is hard to tell whether it will grow back or not. If you have had gradual thinning and then it suddenly sheds much more, this is not likely to be merely telogen effluvium. On the other hand, if you have always had a full head of hair and notice an increase in shedding, it is reasonable to wait and see if the hair will grow back. Events that induce shedding include childbirth, surgery with general anesthesia, and a fever higher than 101 to 102 degrees for more than a day or so. Flu does not ordinarily cause later hair loss. Most women, however, will experience shedding after having a baby or after general anesthesia. The shedding does not occur right away, because after the hairs enter the inactive telogen phase, they remain on the scalp for several weeks before falling out. Because of this delay, it is often almost impossible to figure out what might have caused hair loss. Commonly, whatever external factor triggered the hair loss has been completely forgotten by the time the shedding occurs.

External factors such as hair-care preparations do not seem to be important as causes of hair loss. They may not always make hair look as good as they say they will, but they are unlikely to damage your hair.

Nutrition is not usually a factor in androgenic alopecia. Many people believe that if their hair or fingernails are weak the problem may be poor nutrition. It is true that hair is a protein and that lack of protein in famine conditions results in hair that is discolored and brittle. This is not seen in the United States or other developed countries unless the malnutrition is caused by an illness. Very strict diets or anorexia nervosa can result in hair loss. If the dieting does not continue too long—say, several months—the hair usually grows back. Zinc deficiency is thought to be associated with alopecia, and some doctors recommend supplements. There is nothing wrong with this practice so long as excessive doses are not taken. However, zinc deficiency is usually not the fundamental problem. I would not recommend depending solely on zinc supplements because they are not likely to help you.

It will probably seem strange to you that androgens can inhibit hair growth since they also cause too much of it. Androgens stimulate growth of hair on the face and the body but cause loss of hair from the scalp. The extreme of this is seen in men who have less scalp hair and more hair everywhere else, compared to women. Hair follicles on the scalp respond to androgens but in a different way than those on the face or body. Instead of becoming more active, they become less so.

I have referred to the effect of testosterone in androgenic alopecia as inactivating the hair follicle because this is what seems to happen. Although everyone refers to "losing" hair, actually it is not really lost. The follicle is still there but is so inactive that it produces only a fine vellus hair that is so small as to be nearly invisible. The fact that there is still a hair growing gives hope that treatment might be possible, although after many years there does seem to be loss of follicles also.

Some women I see have been told that their hair loss is "genetic." An alternative term for androgenic alopecia is "androgenetic" alopecia, to stress that it results from a combination of genetic factors and androgen hormones. This is correct so far as it goes. The tendency for a hair follicle to be vulnerable to inactivation by androgens is inherited, although it does not necessarily affect every family member. Some women I see tell me their mothers have very thin hair, and some notice very early thinning in their teenage or young adult daughters. If one or more female relatives have alopecia, it is more likely but not certain that you will develop it also.

It is a common misconception that if a condition is genetic nothing can be done about it. Genetic does not mean untreatable. A good example is correction of subnormal height with growth hormone. It was once thought that if someone was very short and had short parents growth hormone would not work. This has turned out not to be the case at all.

Treatment of Androgenic Alopecia

Diagnostic testing for androgenic alopecia is the same as for hirsutism and acne, and so is interpretation of results. Tests show which hormones are elevated—total and free testosterone, androstenedione, DHEA-S, or a combination. The same dex test can distinguish whether the problem is in the ovary or the adrenal gland. The majority of women with androgenic alopecia actually do not have elevated androgen levels but have increased sensitivity of their hair follicles to androgens. Some who have normal androgens may have had higher levels a few years earlier. Even though the levels go down, the inactivation of hair follicles continues. Of course, some with alopecia do have high androgens. If early changes of menopause are a possibility, estradiol and FSH are measured.

Alopecia is a gradual process; it takes many years of exposure to androgens before scalp hair follicles become inactive. And some women with very thick hair do not notice any change until the process has been going on for several years.

Treatments for androgenic alopecia are really the same as treatments for other kinds of androgenic disorders, which I explained in detail in the previous chapter. An anti-androgen such as spironolactone or flutamide is used. The recently introduced drug finasteride may help alopecia but is unproven. Lowering androgen levels by birth control pills or dexamethasone may also be necessary, but by itself will not help alopecia.

The first effect of treatment is that shedding slows down and the hair becomes healthier and livelier-looking. It looks fuller even if no more hairs have appeared. These improvements can usually be noticed in the first few weeks on medication, assuming that the right medicines were chosen for you. If shedding is not better by three to four months of treatment, adjustment of medication has to be considered. Regrowth, if it is to occur, usually does not begin until the second year of treatment. If your shedding slows to normal, this is a good sign. Be patient because there is a good chance that you will eventually have at least some regrowth. The response of alopecia to treatment is slow because hair growth is a slow process. Not all physicians believe that endocrine treatment is effective for alopecia. I think one reason is that they do not realize how long it takes to work.

It is hard to tell what percentage of women treated for androgenic alopecia have regrowth. Many do, but certainly not all. However, treatment is almost always successful in arresting progression. The shorter the time alopecia has been present, the greater the likelihood that there will be regrowth with treatment. If you have the problem, I suggest you seek out help now rather than wait years to see what will happen.

I've mentioned that not all hair loss is permanent. Sometimes women are told by a dermatologist or other doctor that their hair loss is telogen effluvium and will eventually all grow back. When I first became interested in hormonal hair disorders, I marveled at how a doctor could tell when hair loss was temporary and when it was permanent. Finally I realized that usually one cannot tell. Sometimes a woman will have a period of rapid shedding (telogen effluvium) without any event clearly causing it, and it will grow back. More often it is just the early stages of androgenic or estrogen-deficiency alopecia. My advice is that, unless you have had one of the events I mentioned earlier, if you begin losing hair, have it evaluated.

Estrogen Deficiency and Alopecia

The treatments I have discussed are aimed at lowering androgen levels or blocking their effects on the hair and skin. However, many women have alopecia that results not from anything to do with androgens but from falling levels of estrogen. While the fall in estrogen after giving birth is the cause of the shedding many women have a few weeks later, the hair usually grows back in the ensuing months. When hair loss occurs due to falling estrogen levels with menopause, it will not grow back on its own. It is not unusual to have hair loss as one of the earliest signs of menopause, before periods stop. Many women come to me because they have started to lose their hair but had not realized any connection to menopause. Hair loss is a part of menopause that has not received much emphasis, either from the medical profession or in the lay press. This is unfortunate because of all forms of alopecia, it responds best to treatment.

As I explained earlier, estrogen-deficiency alopecia does not look different from androgenic alopecia and is not distinguished in textbooks. So far as I know, I was the first to recognize it as having a cause distinct from that of androgenic alopecia. Clues that estrogen deficiency is what is causing hair loss are the age at which it began, the presence of other menopausal symptoms, and lab results. Usually in this form of alopecia, all sex steroids are low, androgens and estrogens both.

Treatment is simple because it consists of estrogen replacement. There are other important health reasons why you may want to choose to take estrogen replacement; these are discussed in Chapter Thirteen. The minimum doses of estrogen that are sufficient to decrease the risk of osteoporosis and heart disease usually will not stop alopecia very effectively. The hair follicles simply need more estrogen than the bones and blood vessels. However, the emphasis currently in treatment of menopause is on decreasing the risk of later disease rather than on present well-being. I expect that this situation will change as more and more doctors become more expert in treating estrogen deficiency.

Estrogen replacement is discussed in complete detail in Chapter Thirteen. Here I will simply repeat what doses usually work best for alopecia. For conjugated estrogens (Premarin®) or estrone (Ogen®, Abbot), 1.25 mg daily is more likely to be effective than the more common doses of 0.625. For micronized estradiol (Estrace®), there is less information, but usually 2 or 3 mg daily is needed. For the skin patch (Estraderm®, Ciba-Geigy), it is the larger size, 0.1 mg. Sometimes slightly higher doses than those I have just stated are needed. The question of proper use of estrogen is an important one for all women, and I recommend that you read the chapter on that subject.

Care of the Hair and Scalp

If you are losing hair, it is natural to wonder if it is due to the hair-care products you are using. While the situation was different several decades ago when there were many dangerous cosmetic products around, this is rarely the case now. Regulation by the FDA is more stringent, and companies do not want to risk their reputation or incur lawsuits by selling products that are harmful. Consumers are now very alert to any ill effects of products they use. In general, it is best to stick to products made by the large, well-established companies. They test their products very carefully; smaller ones may not be able to afford to. Laws are not as strict in some other countries; if you have a hair problem, it may be prudent to take along a supply of the products that work for you when you travel.

Shampoos rarely cause problems; at worst, they can dry hair or leave it too oily, resulting in a look you are not happy with. In neither case is the hair follicle affected. If your hair tends to seem dry and brittle after shampooing or is hard to comb, the answer is not to stop washing your hair but to use conditioner. Once you find what works for you, stay with it. There is no truth in the idea that it is better for your hair to change shampoos from time to time.

Many women with alopecia want to perm their hair. This may make your hair cover your scalp better. Perms are usually not harmful; however, to be sure, ask your hairdresser to be sure to do a complete neutralization step. While the chemicals used in perms generally do not damage hair, rolling the hair tight can. Use fairly wide rollers and settle for loose curls.

Dyeing has more potential to damage hair than do perms. Washable or semi-permanent dyes are unlikely to damage hair, but permanent ones can. Bleaching is hard on hair, and coloring methods that require bleaching first are most damaging. It is always safer to make your hair darker rather than lighter.

On the other hand, dark hair may make alopecia more apparent because of the contrast with the skin of the scalp. Recently, dark-colored hair sprays have become available that temporarily darken the scalp so as to make thin hair less conspicuous. An advantage of dyeing is that the hair becomes a little fluffier because of the effects of the dye on the hair shaft. Henna itself is very damaging, but most henna products use modified forms that are safe. If you have hair problems, it is best not to have your hair dyed and permed at the same time. Have the perm first, and go back to have it dyed a week or two later when your hair has recovered.

In the past, hair-straightening methods for black women sometimes employed lye, which is very damaging to hair. Newer ones have no lye and are much safer. Some black hair styles require pulling the hair to braid it or sweep it back. This can pull hair out by the roots unless it is done very gently. Areas of thin hair around braids are almost always due to this traction alopecia. Pomade in the hair makes it worse because the hair sticks together and is more likely to come out when pulled back.

Some home-styling practices can damage hair or pull it out. One of the most common is something you may have been told as a child was good for your hair: brushing it. The bristles catch the hair and are much more likely to pull it out than the teeth of a comb. If you have alopecia, do not brush your hair. If it is tangled, comb it out slowly, a short distance at a time. Use of a blow-dryer in itself is not harmful to hair, but heat makes the hair brittle; the combination of combing and hot blow-drying is a bad one. I suggest you buy a blow-dryer that allows you to turn the heat down. Blow-drying this way takes longer but will not cause your hair to break off.

None of the practices I have been warning about here will affect hair-growth mechanisms. A bad dye or perm might leave your hair looking less attractive or cause it to break off or, in the worst case, pull it out by the root. But none will permanently damage the follicle so that it cannot grow a new hair. Damage will eventually disappear when new hair has replaced the old. However, since this takes many months, it is best to keep your hair in good shape to begin with.

Some women have seborrhea of the scalp with their alopecia. This is similar to seborrhea of the face. It is a condition in which extra sebum (oil) is being produced in response to androgens. The most common sign is dandruff, in which the bits of skin that normally fall off unnoticed stick to the hair and scalp because of the oiliness. Itching is another symptom. In more severe cases, there may be crusting on the scalp and sometimes even infection. Anti-androgen therapy works best, but a good anti-seborrhea shampoo helps a lot. Neutragena T-Gel® is excellent. A stronger version is T-Sel®. If you have scalp seborrhea, you should wash with a suitable shampoo, generally once a day. If your hair is dried out by this, use a conditioner or alternate with a milder shampoo. A topical glucocorticoid cream or lotion can help if crusts are stubborn.

Minoxidil (Rogaine®, Upjohn) is the medication best known for treating alopecia. Although it is a prescription drug that has been advertised on television and in magazines, it has not become very widely used.

Originally minoxidil was introduced for treatment of high blood pressure. It was soon noticed that both men and women taking this drug began to experience hair growth where they had none before, such as the forehead. Because of this side effect, it is rarely used as an antihypertensive today. Since there was no way to control *where* the hair appeared on those who were taking it, it was of no use for treating hair loss. However, a topical preparation was developed that could be applied only to the skin area on which more hair was wanted: the scalp. The current preparation contains a 2 percent solution of minoxidil, and a stronger 4 percent solution is being developed.

Minoxidil has been far less popular among both men and women than its manufacturer had hoped. There are several problems with it in actual use. Only about a third of the people using it get *any* increase in their hair, and for many of these the increase is not enough to make the treatment worth the effort and expense. Minoxidil must be applied to the entire scalp twice a day, which is time consuming and may affect the appearance of the hair, and it is also expensive: about $55 per month. Because any hair that grows as a result of minoxidil treatment will be lost if the drug is discontinued, the person starting minoxidil is making a very long-term commitment.

Most of the women I have treated with minoxidil have not been satisfied with the results, and eventually discontinued using it. It seems to be most satisfactory when a limited area of hair loss—such as the small areas of thinning hair which many women experience on their temples—is not fully responding to hormonal treatment. When only a small area needs to be treated, the inconvenience and cost are much less.

I do not recommend that you start minoxidil at the same time as other treatments, because if your hair improves you will not know whether it is the minoxidil or the other medication which has helped and you may feel obligated to continue both.

The advantage of minoxidil is that it does not require hormonal testing or an endocrinologist to be prescribed. If you cannot get advice in your area regarding other treatments, you may decide minoxidil is worth a try. If you do try it, be patient because it takes about nine months to see any improvement.

A stronger form of minoxidil is being studied and will probably be introduced in a few years. There are also studies of combinations of minoxidil with other medications applied to the scalp. It is possible that these new forms will be more effective than the present one.

Alopecia Areata

One morning when Angela woke up, she noticed a bunch of hairs on her pillow, almost as if she had been cutting her hair and failed to clean up the hairs. Surprised, she felt around on her scalp, but her hair was all there, or so it seemed. She next went into the bathroom and looked in the mirror. At first glance, she noticed nothing amiss. But then, as she held up her hair in various areas so as to be able to see her scalp, she found an area behind her left ear that was bare of hair. It was only about an inch in diameter and could only be seen when the rest of the hair around it was picked up. Angela at first thought that she might have done something injurious to her scalp or hair, but she could not recollect anything. A few days later, the spot was larger, and two weeks later she found another area in which her scalp showed because the hair was gone. This was on top, slightly to the right side. It could be covered by other hair but was not as completely hidden as the other spot.

It was a month later that Angela came to see me and told me the story. She was about to turn twenty-eight and worked as a receptionist in an advertising agency. She told me that she had always thought her striking long black hair was her best feature and that she'd been "in a panic that it's all about to fall out." Appearance was particularly important in the field she worked in; although she didn't really think she'd lose her job, she felt very uncomfortable. "I'm not ready at twenty-seven to start wearing a wig." Everything else about Angela was normal. I found nothing suggestive of ill health in her medical history and her physical exam was also entirely normal.

Angela did not have androgenic alopecia. Rather she had a condition known as alopecia areata. This is very different from androgenic alopecia. (Remember, alopecia is just a general term meaning hair loss. There are many forms of alopecia.) Alopecia areata is not a hormonal disorder at all, although very rarely it can be found together with underactivity of the thyroid, parathyroid, adrenal, or pituitary gland.

Alopecia areata is caused by a disorder of the immune system and is a form of autoimmune disease. Autoimmune diseases occur when the body's immune system attacks normal body tissue. The most complex aspect of immune function is how the body distinguishes "self"—that is, normal tissue that belongs in the body—from "nonself," foreign or harmful tissue such as viruses or bacteria. Because the differences between self and nonself are so subtle, it is not surprising that sometimes the immune system fails to realize that certain tissues are self and attacks them. Some tissues are more likely to undergo autoimmune attack than others. In general, women are more susceptible to autoimmune problems than men. A woman's immune system is more complex than a man's because it needs to have a special mechanism so that during pregnancy it does not turn against the baby she is carrying.

In alopecia areata, the immune system attacks the hair follicles as if they were foreign tissue and needed to be destroyed. A biopsy of the scalp shows immunologically active cells surrounding the hair follicles. What starts the immune attack on the hair follicle in alopecia areata is unknown. The course is unpredictable also. Usually the hair grows back within a few months, but sometimes the condition progresses and other areas lose their hair. Even when the hair grows back, there are often future episodes, equally sudden and unexplained.

Alopecia areata can be accompanied by a skin disorder known as vitiligo. This is the loss of pigment from a discrete area with relatively distinct borders. It is also autoimmune, but what is destroyed by the immune system is not hair follicles but pigmentary cells. Like alopecia areata, vitiligo is sometimes found with more serious autoimmune disease of the internal organs or endocrine glands. Other than these associations with other disease, vitiligo is harmless, though the loss of pigmentation is often visible and embarrassing. The most common place for it to occur is the hands and forearms. Often both sides are affected in a somewhat symmetrical manner. The face can also be affected. People with dark pigmentation, such as blacks, Asians, and Mediterraneans, have the hardest time with vitiligo because there is greater contrast between the very pale skin that has lost its pigment and the normal dark skin. In very fair whites, vitiligo may be almost invisible. Sometimes it becomes noticeable only in summertime, when the normal skin tans and the vitiligo-affected skin does not. There are treatments for vitiligo that are partially effective. I will not cover them here because vitiligo is really a skin disorder, not a hormonal one. I have mentioned it because it sometimes accompanies autoimmune diseases of the endocrine system.

Please be reassured that, while I have seen many women with both conditions, I have not seen anyone in whom alopecia areata or vitiligo was the first sign of more serious autoimmune disease. Nor have I ever seen a woman who had only alopecia areata or vitiligo go on to develop more serious autoimmune disease. When autoimmune disease is present there are other signs. If you have either condition, medical evaluation is advisable, but you have no need to feel very anxious.

The most common hormonal problem associated with alopecia areata is a thyroid disorder called Hashimoto's thyroiditis, an inflammatory condition. There is no pain, but the thyroid gland gradually loses its ability to function. It is very much like alopecia areata except that the immune system is attacking the thyroid. Hashimoto's thyroiditis is very common in women, affecting 1 to 3 percent. If you have alopecia areata, your chance of having or developing Hashimoto's thyroiditis is increased. You should have your thyroid evaluated by physical examination; you should have initial blood tests and then repeat them every two to four years. The most that can happen with Hashimoto's is that your thyroid will become underactive. This can be treated simply, easily, and cheaply with thyroid medication. If you are properly treated for it, your metabolism will be entirely normal. You will be equally healthy whether your body gets its thyroid hormone from your thyroid gland or from a pill.

Symptoms of an underactive thyroid gland are sluggishness, fatigue, depression, and weight gain, though only mild weight gain can be attributed to a thyroid condition. Sometimes it can cause generalized puffiness, especially noticeable around the eyes in women in their fifties or older. All these symptoms sound common, and they are. Most women who feel tired or puffy do not have hypothyroidism. Plain depression and weight gain due to a change in diet or exercise are far more common. (See Chapters Eight, Nine, and Ten.)

Hypothyroidism is easily overlooked because the symptoms are common and not specific to thyroid disease. If you have these symptoms, you should certainly have your thyroid checked. But if adequate testing shows your thyroid to be normal, it is more worthwhile to look elsewhere for an explanation. There have been great advances in thyroid testing in the last decade, and any degree of hypothyroidism can be detected with the newer tests.

Autoimmunity can damage the ovary, although this is rare. If all you have is vitiligo or alopecia, then you need not worry about this condition.

Changes in hair or skin are often imagined to be a sign of general ill health. This is not really true. Rather these conditions are alarming because they can be seen. With the exceptions I have discussed, alopecia areata and vitiligo are not signs of being unhealthy. Nor are they related to nutrition any more than is androgenic alopecia.

Let's return to Angela's story. Hers is rather typical of mild or early alopecia areata. Hair loss began suddenly. Everything was fine until one morning she found that an area of her scalp had lost all its hair. (This is the source of the name areata; hair is lost from distinct areas.) This area enlarged, and then a new area of hair loss appeared. Angela was relatively fortunate. She had only two areas of hair loss, and both were small enough to be covered by other hair. The main problem for Angela was worrying about what would happen to her hair in the future.

I was able to reassure her only partially. For the vast majority of women who have an episode of alopecia areata, the lost hair all grows back and the episode is all but forgotten. I was able to tell Angela that this was the most likely outcome. But I also had to tell her that there was a possibility that hair loss would recur and that there would be one or more future episodes. Angela's hair did grow back by itself, but she did have another episode two years later involving a different, smaller area. This hair grew back also. That was five years ago; so far as I know she has had no more problems.

Other women with alopecia areata are not always as fortunate as Angela. In some, the area of loss enlarges, and a substantial portion of the scalp becomes bare. The edges of the scalp are more often affected than the top. This is one of the ways alopecia areata can be distinguished from androgenic alopecia. In the latter, the top is most affected, and the sides never lose all their hair. Women with androgenic alopecia almost never lose all their hair; there are always some strands on the thinnest areas. In contrast, alopecia areata usually results in loss of all hair in an affected area. If the area involved is small, then alopecia areata is less visible to others than androgenic alopecia, but large areas are harder to hide.

More extreme forms of alopecia areata are called alopecia areata totalis and alopecia areata universalis. In the totalis form, all the hairs of the scalp are lost, as well as eyebrow and eyelash hair. This is quite different from androgenic alopecia, which involves only the scalp. In the universalis form, all or nearly all body hair is lost, including pubic, underarm, and leg hair. The distinction between these forms is not absolute. Some women with only partial hair loss on their scalp will notice some mild thinning of the eyelashes or body hair. Thinning of some areas of body hair is not unusual for women over time; by itself it does not usually mean that any more severe or noticeable hair thinning will develop.

To treat alopecia areata, it is necessary to suppress the immune system. Unfortunately all drugs that do this have significant hazards or side effects. The ones most commonly used are prednisone or related glucocorticoids. Prednisone can be free of side effects in tiny doses, but the higher doses necessary to suppress the immune system always have side effects. The most disturbing to woman who must take it, though not necessarily the most serious, is weight gain. Their effect on how one looks is not a flattering one. I do not recommend using oral prednisone or other glucocorticoids for alopecia areata. If you are considering this form of treatment, I recommend that you read my discussion of them in Chapter Two.

There is one way glucocorticoids can be used safely for alopecia areata—by injection under the scalp of the affected areas. (Just applying it onto the skin does not work because it does not get all the way down into the hair follicles.) A variety of potent synthetic glucocorticoids are used for this purpose. All have been in use for a long time and are safe when used in moderate doses. Triamcinolone (Kenalog®, Westwood-Squibb) is one such injectable medication, but there are many others. The choice should be left to the dermatologist who is doing the procedure. The basic limitation of intralesional injection, as this is called, is that it is just not practical if large areas are affected, because of pain and the large total dose that would be required. My suggestion, if you have developed alopecia areata, is that you first wait a few months. Often the hair will all grow back. If this does not seem to be happening, consult a dermatologist and consider having injections of glucocorticoid into the lesion. If a large amount of hair has been lost, you may want to seek medical evaluation sooner.

Chapter Eight

•

Fluid Retention:
Puffiness and Bloating

*F*rom time immemorial, water has been a symbol of femininity. The psychologist Carl Jung included water in his idea of the feminine archetype. In Chinese philosophy, yin, the feminine principle present in all things, includes dampness. The sea is also symbolic of women, in part because, to men at least, women seem mysterious, like the ocean depths.

The tides, one of the most basic and powerful rhythms of nature, are controlled by the moon, which is also a feminine symbol. Because the full cycle of moon and tides is twenty-eight days, about the same as the length of the menstrual cycle, there is a mythic as well as a physiological association between the menstrual cycle and fluid shifts. There is a tendency to associate changes in body water with the menstrual cycle and to look at them as powerful natural forces that greatly affect a woman's life. While the moon is a feminine symbol, it is also associated with strangeness and ill luck. Abnormal behavior was once explained as due to a full moon. The words "lunacy" and "lunatic" refer to the ancient attribution of mental abnormality to effects of the moon. Changes in water, the menstrual cycle, and mood changes seem interconnected.

In the ancient world, women and men conceived of the body as a universe in miniature. This idea manifests itself in astrology, which is basically a belief in the correspondence between heavenly bodies and our own lives. Because the moon is not so obvious from the city night as it must have been to primitive women and men, we are less inclined to observe it and relate it directly to our moods and lives. But the idea that something external controls the watery part of the body is still very much present.

There are other associations between femininity and water. Emotion in women is expressed through water, both the tears of mental or physical pain and the hidden moisture of sexual arousal. Hormones themselves, so important in a woman's life, are carried in the water of the blood. Babies are protected by the water of the amniotic fluid while being carried in their mothers' bodies. In the breasts is formed the fluid that provides nourishment for the newborn baby. Internal water is part of the physical nurturing function of a woman's body. Indeed premenstrual water retention is part of the preparation of a woman's body for pregnancy, which begins anew every month with the luteal phase of her cycle.

Fluid changes seem mysterious. Fluid in the body can be felt in the form of swelling, but it cannot be seen directly. Fluid retention seems to be a powerful force intervening in a woman's life. Water can greatly affect the way a woman feels and what clothes she can wear.

Consider Elizabeth, an immaculately groomed forty-two-year-old whose husband is a prominent businessman in a midwestern city. Elizabeth had worked as an administrative secretary prior to having children. Now that her children were in high school and college, she spent her time working with various charitable organizations. This, as well as her husband's business, required a considerable amount of socializing. These demands had become a strain for her because of the problem she had consulted me about: fluid retention associated with her menstrual cycle. Elizabeth explained to me she had so much swelling and bloating that she needed two separate wardrobes; also she was very embarrassed to have her swollen ankles show during the week before her period. Since there were many rather formal events in her social schedule, this presented quite a problem for her.

Her internist had prescribed a water pill, hydrochlorothiazide (Hydrodiuril®, Merck); while this had helped at first, the swelling was now worse, despite the medication. Elizabeth had become very depressed about the situation. She hoped that an endocrinologist could explain why she was having so much fluid retention and find a way to correct the hormonal imbalance she thought must be causing it. After doing her physical, which showed signs of mild fluid retention in her legs, I ordered some tests and arranged for a follow-up visit in two weeks. That night I got a call from the laboratory because her potassium was so low that it was flagged by the computer as possibly dangerous. This did not entirely surprise me because low potassium is a common complication of the overuse of diuretics like hydrochlorothiazide.

Elizabeth had a condition called idiopathic cyclic edema, which is simply the extreme form of the premenstrual fluid retention that causes discomfort to millions of women. ("Idiopathic" simply means that the cause is unknown.)

Fluid and Mood

Some patients and some doctors attribute all the unpleasant effects of premenstrual syndrome (PMS) to fluid retention. Prominent in PMS are depression and a certain kind of irritability in which a woman may feel angry at her children, husband, and others who are close or important to her. Some women fear that these relationships may be damaged by their angry behavior at these times. As one of my patients told me, "Finally my husband gently pointed out that he was great for two weeks out of the month and terrible for the other two weeks and that maybe the difference was in my hormones rather than in him." This is one of the worst parts of PMS for many women: the difficulty in telling whether the irritation or hurt feelings of this time are justified or just a peculiar by-product of shifting waters and hormones. It is hard to try to work out the problems of a relationship when you are uncertain as to whether they are real or imagined. Of course, women with PMS can have justified complaints in a relationship, and men have been known to use PMS as a way of discrediting the concerns of their wives or girlfriends. More innocently, they also can be simply confused by the cyclic changes in a woman's body.

Feeling swollen is uncomfortable, and this may make one feel irritable or mildly depressed. But fluid retention is not the only cause of PMS. Some women have mood changes without any fluid retention, and others get puffy without being sensitive or sad. Fluid retention and PMS overlap but are not identical.

Water and the Body

In order to better understand female fluid problems and how they can be helped, it is helpful to consider water in the body from a scientific point of view. About 55 to 60 percent of the human body is water. Water is necessary for life because the chemical reactions that constitute life can go on only in a solution. There is no life form that is dry. The body must regulate everything concerning water with great exactitude.

The body must control two things about water: its distribution and its concentration. The distribution of water goes awry in fluid retention. Water oozes out of the blood vessels and into the loose tissue under the skin. The medical term for the presence of extra water in the tissues of the body is *edema*. Edema can occur anywhere from the brain on down and has many different causes.

The kind of edema that women experience with hormonal conditions is influenced by gravity, which causes most of it to accumulate at the lowest parts of the body: the feet, ankles, and lower legs. These parts are also farthest from the heart, so they have the least efficient circulation. One result is that when there is extra fluid in the legs, it may take a long time to get rid of it. It is also harder for your blood vessels to reabsorb fluid if you are overweight, because the extra fat increases the pressure pushing the fluid out of the circulation into the soft tissues of the legs. Prolonged standing increases the amount of the body's fluid that goes to the legs. However, exercise involving the legs, like jogging, eases edema as the contraction of the muscles helps to pump the fluid out of the legs. Inactivity is the worst thing for fluid retention. Edema can also affect the thighs and waist, but usually not nearly as much as the lower legs. Edema means swelling and weight gain; shoes and pants are suddenly too tight. The weight of the water shows up on the scale. In a culture where controlling weight is a struggle for so many, an extra pound is never welcome, even if it is water rather than fat.

Edema is too much water in the wrong places. To understand why it gets there, you must consider the other important thing about water in the body: its concentration. The amount of water relative to the things dissolved in it, especially salt, must be maintained within very narrow limits. If there is not enough water, the cells dry out, taking on a shrunken appearance under a microscope. If there is too much water in a cell, it swells. Cells, as well as ankles, can have edema. Water tends to move to where dissolved chemicals are more concentrated. This process, called osmosis, causes water to tend to even out its distribution throughout the body. If there is too much water in the circulation, it travels out of the blood vessels and ends up under the skin.

Sodium is the main chemical that maintains adequate water in the cells of the body. (Often the terms "sodium" and "salt" are used interchangeably, even though salt contains chloride as well as sodium. For our purposes, the terms are synonymous because the important part of salt is sodium.) Wherever there is extra sodium in the body, water eventually follows, to reduce the sodium concentration to normal. This is why salt starts the process of fluid retention. When we take in more salt, we need more water to maintain the two in normal balance. The fluid retention experienced is unpleasant, but less so than the changes in the body that would result from having relatively more salt than water. Eventually, if one is healthy, the body gets rid of the extra salt as well as the extra water. Then fluid retention goes away. The problem with this process is that it may take several days, during which there is still discomfort from fluid retention. One reason the process can be slow is that certain hormones may try to get the body to hold on to both the salt and the water.

When less salt is taken in, the body lets go of more water. This is why the best way to prevent fluid retention is to take in as little salt as possible. While our bodies do need some salt, our food contains so much of it that we do not need to add any. Diuretics can deplete the body of salt as well as potassium and other essential elements.

You do need to have enough water in your body; there must be enough for the circulation to function efficiently. The blood must carry oxygen and all other important substances to the tissues. To do so, there must be an adequate volume of blood. Mild decrease in the volume of fluid in the circulation is common and shows itself by such familiar symptoms as dizziness or feeling faint when standing up. Everyone has experienced these, for example, as a result of exercising in the summer's heat. The loss of water through sweating causes a very slight decrease in the volume of the blood.

We are totally dependent on the circulatory system for survival, and so the body has very exacting mechanisms for holding on to salt and water. However, a consequence of the vigor of these mechanisms is that sometimes they function more strongly than they need to. Hormones regulate the amount of water in the body, but their main function is to maintain enough water within the circulation so that blood will continue to flow through the tissues. It is the amount of water in the circulation that these hormones regulate best, not the amount in the places women do not want water, like their ankles and legs. Your body would rather err on the side of retaining too much water than risk a decrease in blood volume.

Salt, Water, and the Menstrual Cycle

To consider why the premenstrual state is associated with fluid retention in many women, we must introduce another major action of the hormone progesterone, which rises to very high levels in the second two weeks of the cycle. Progesterone relaxes the smooth muscle of the uterus so that it will not contract and expel the developing baby. It also acts on other smooth muscle and has the same effect. This causes the intestinal smooth muscle to relax and expand, accounting for the abdominal bloating that is another premenstrual symptom. It also causes the smooth muscle around the arteries to relax. Because there is more space in the blood vessels when their walls relax, the body needs to increase the volume of the blood. It does this by releasing aldosterone from the adrenal gland and vasopressin from the pituitary gland, which causes to kidney to hold onto more sodium and water. Some of this water stays in the circulation, but some filters out into the tissues.

Late in the cycle of many women, the body retains more

salt and water than it needs to. If pregnancy occurred during this cycle, the retention of water and sodium would be needed in preparing the body to support the developing child. Here evolution seems to have been more concerned to equip women to carry on the species than to be comfortable. Fortunately medicine provides at least some help in overcoming this situation.

Fluid Retention
Apart from the Menstrual Cycle

Men can have water retention, too, although most never experience it unless they have heart, liver, or kidney disease. In certain circumstances, the male hormone testosterone can produce fluid retention. Testosterone is anabolic; it helps the body form new tissue or repair old tissue. Since at least 60 percent of the body is water, for new tissue to be formed the body must retain water. It also must retain sodium, also an essential part of new tissue, so that the two will be in balance. Anything, therefore, that promotes new tissue formation will have the potential to produce water retention. Usually at puberty, the rise in testosterone is so gradual that no edema is noticed. However, when given to teens or men who have a deficiency, testosterone can cause very noticeable water retention, with swelling of the ankles and legs and puffiness of the hands. This problem can be prevented by starting with a low dose and increasing it gradually, giving the body time to use the water for the growing muscles rather than depositing it in the soft tissue of the legs. Insulin is another anabolic hormone. It promotes the use of food—sugar, protein, and fat—to make new tissue. Without insulin, the body cannot use these nutrients efficiently, which is why sugar is lost in the urine when people have diabetes. Insulin can cause edema in certain circumstances.

There are several diseases that can cause edema. In congestive heart failure, a condition in which the heart is no longer able to power the circulation, the heart cannot fully pump out all the blood returning to it. This causes pressure to build up in the circulatory system, which in turn causes water to ooze out of the capillaries and into the tissues. The result is edema. In some kidney conditions, the kidney cannot get rid of extra water and edema also forms. Liver disease can produce pressure changes within the circulation in the abdomen, causing water to ooze into the abdominal cavity. The result is swelling of the abdomen.

You may hear of these situations or come across them in other reading. These are uncommon situations, and invariably other symptoms are present before the water retention becomes severe. The woman with swollen ankles need not be worried that she has heart, kidney, or liver disease, especially if a tendency to swelling has been a long-time problem. But the sudden appearance of a great deal of fluid retention should prompt medical evaluation.

What Can Be Done to Help Fluid Retention—and What Should Not Be Done

Fluid retention is not hopeless. Certain things can be done to help, and they do make a difference. Taking medications is usually not a good answer. Treatment for fluid retention employs diuretics, a class of drugs that help the body rid itself of salt and water. Most of the popular ones, such as chlorothiazide (Diuril®, Merck), hydrochlorothiazide (Hydrodiuril®, Merck), and furosemide (Lasix®, Hoechst Roussel), act by preventing the kidney from reabsorbing sodium during the process of urine formation. As we have seen, water follows salt and so water is lost as well.

All these diuretics, and furosemide in particular, are quite effective in increasing excretion of water from the body, with a great increase in urination being noticed quite quickly. A modest amount of leg edema can be removed completely by one or two doses of furosemide.

Unfortunately, diuretics present two problems. First, they increase not only water and sodium loss but also the loss of other minerals as well. Potassium deficiency will occur after only one or two doses of furosemide. Other minerals are also lost, notably magnesium. Some doctors believe that magnesium deficiency is common and can cause chronic fatigue.

There is no question but that low potassium levels cause fatigue and weakness. If potassium gets very low, fatal changes in heart rhythm can occur. A low potassium level is a serious situation. Elizabeth had potassium deficiency as a result of taking furosemide. Some of the fatigue and generally not feeling well, which she had assumed were also due to her fluid retention, were actually due to the long-standing potassium deficiency induced by the diuretic. If you are taking any of the three diuretics I have mentioned, you need to be on either a potassium supplement or another medication to help your body keep its potassium.

The other serious problem with diuretics is that they can be addicting. We have seen that edema occurs because certain hormones behave as if the body were short of water. Diuretics get it to pour out water despite this. But, once the diuretic has worn off, the body notices that it has even less water and the processes that caused salt and water retention to begin with go into overdrive. The result is even more fluid retention. This is not too severe if only two or three doses have been taken. But if diuretic use is more prolonged, they can make fluid retention much worse. As soon as the diuretic is discontinued, the body does what it wanted to do in the first place: retain water. A vicious cycle occurs in which the problem of fluid retention is not solved but hidden. The rebound edema after discontinuation of diuretics is usually worse than the mild edema that was the reason for trying diuretics in the first place. The more potent the diuretic, the greater is the edema on its discontinuation. Furosemide is the worst in this respect. If they are stopped, which they should be, a period of more severe fluid retention, with worse discomfort, begins and may last two or more weeks before the extra fluid is finally lost.

If you begin to rely on diuretics to get rid of excess fluid, you may find yourself in a situation where you feel you need to take them all the time, and you may end up taking higher and higher doses. This is a situation not unlike an addiction, although diuretics are certainly not harmful in the way alcohol, cocaine, or opiates are. Women who are very concerned about their weight are sometimes tempted to take diuretics. Women with anorexia nervosa or bulimia commonly use them. The reason is that water is heavy and someone who uses a diuretic and then steps on the scale a few hours later will notice a decrease of several pounds. The weight loss is quite useless because what is lost is not fat but water, and water loss does nothing for appearance and even less for health. But, with the obsession about weight in our culture, some people become focused on the scale and what it shows. Being of normal weight is positive, but when the pursuit of low weight as measured on the scale becomes self-perpetuating without reference to health, feeling well, or being attractive, it has a decidedly negative effect on one's life. If you find yourself starting to try to control your weight with diuretics, you may need to seek professional counseling.

How is it possible to get off diuretics if one is unfortunate enough to have become habituated to them? First, a high degree of determination is necessary, because there will be some uncomfortable days. It is best to choose a time when other stresses can be minimized: a vacation, a slow period at work, certainly a time free of special occasions, such as weddings or class reunions, when you may be particularly concerned about how you look. The help of an experienced, supportive doctor is invaluable. The dose should be gradually reduced by either decreasing the daily amount or by spreading out doses to every two and then every three days. Within two weeks, however, the diuretics should be stopped. Tapering for too long a time merely prolongs the misery. Three weeks may be required for the rebound edema to go away. Be reassured, however, that it always does go away.

Diuretics are not very harmful if used with restraint. A safe maximum is two, or at most three, doses per cycle. The temptation to use more must be resisted. Furosemide is extremely potent and is meant for patients with severe heart or kidney disease. When used for cyclic edema, it is both dangerous and addicting. Chlorothiazide and hydrochlorothiazide are milder and more appropriate for the healthy woman who tends to retain fluid. They are still strong enough to remove more water than is healthy, especially if they are taken for several days in a row. Because they are potassium-depleting, they are best used in combination with the potassium-sparing drug triamterine as in the combination Dyazide® (SmithKline Beecham) or with a potassium supplement. Spironolactone does not cause rebound edema; while it is a weaker diuretic by itself than the thiazides, it can still be effective for fluid retention. It does not cause the dramatic loss of pounds that the strong diuretics cause, but this is an advantage as its effect on the body is not so drastic. Many women notice a definite improvement in symptoms of PMS with spironolactone. Even if spironolactone is used, the lifestyle measures I describe below are still necessary to overcome fluid retention or PMS.

Preventing Fluid Retention Without Drugs

Measures that are helpful in treating fluid retention are those that tend to limit holding of water in the body and to improve the circulation's ability to reabsorb it from the tissues so the kidneys can get rid of it. The most important step is to lower salt intake to an absolute minimum. Everyone now knows that salt intake can be harmful, but not everyone is aware of what foods are high in salt. It is possible to have a high salt diet without ever picking up a salt shaker. Prepared foods, such as frozen or microwavable dinners, are almost always very high in salt. This is as true of those promoted for weight reduction as it is for the others. The manufacturer has to put some flavor into the food, and the two ready sources are fat and salt.

Some foods that are very high in salt but do not always taste that way are those with tomato sauces or ketchup, including pizza, spaghetti, Mexican food, and fast-food hamburgers. Processed meats contain high amounts of salt, as well as nitrites and other undesirable substances. These include bacon, sausage, luncheon meat, smoked turkey breast, and smoked salmon.

When a woman is in a phase of retaining water and salt, fresh fruit and, especially, vegetables should be chosen in preference to prepared foods. Crisp, fresh vegetables are flavorful, and the lack of salt is not noticed so strongly. With limp, frozen vegetables or boiled ones, the tendency is to try to restore flavor with salt or fat in the form of butter. Chips, salted nuts, and other snack foods are extremely high in both salt and fat.

Some women with fluid problems are overweight. Obesity contributes to fluid retention by increasing the pressure inside the abdomen, which makes it harder for blood to return to the heart. For overweight women who have fluid retention, weight reduction usually cures the problem. I do realize that this is not easy to do; weight reduction is discussed in Chapter

Ten. Anabolic hormones such as insulin tend to promote retention of salt and water because these are essential constituents of new tissue. Carbohydrate, more than fat or protein, stimulates the release of insulin. A decreased carbohydrate intake will result in less need for insulin secretion and less tendency to retain salt and water. Most people who start a diet notice that for a few days they urinate more than usual and that any edema they have is greatly reduced as their weight on the scale decreases. (They are sometimes disappointed that this weight loss does not continue at such a rapid rate once they are rid of the extra fluid.) This tendency for the body to lose fluid when carbohydrate intake is decreased is one of the most useful body mechanisms for a woman with fluid retention. It is nearly impossible to reduce carbohydrate by itself, however, because low carbohydrate foods such as meat or eggs tend to be high in fat, and many are high in salt, too. The only safe way to reduce carbohydrate intake is to reduce total caloric intake.

I am not suggesting anything like a crash diet. Starving one day tends to lead to overeating the next, often of the foods that are least desirable. What is best for fluid retention, if you can do it, is to reduce your food intake by 10 to 20 percent in the days of your cycle in which fluid retention tends to occur. This will make a noticeable difference in how much puffiness you experience. The volume eaten need not decrease if fresh vegetables are substituted for prepared foods that might be eaten at other times. This advice is the sort that is more easily given than followed, but if you can carry it out, it will make a great difference in your well-being. It *may* require changing your routine on those days and preparing different kinds of food for your family as well. It has to be admitted that the same factors induced by progesterone to prepare the body for pregnancy by retaining fluid also tend to stimulate the appetite and sometimes a craving for salt.

You can make your circulatory system more effective, especially in the legs, where fluid tends to accumulate in the greatest amounts. Anything that restricts the return of blood from the legs will make fluid retention worse. This includes tight clothes, upright posture, or sitting for a long time in a cramped position. Airline seats are worst for this, but sitting all day at a desk isn't great either. Keeping your legs elevated will help. Support hose are also effective, but they should be ones like those made by Jobst, which are individually measured so as to fit correctly. Too much tightness at the top of the thigh may make things worse.

Activity of the leg muscles is very important for pumping fluid back into the circulation and up to the heart, where it can be pumped to the kidney to be eliminated. An exercise program will do much to help counteract the tendency for fluid retention, especially aerobic exercise involving the legs. Swimming is best, but running or cycling are also good. Exercise itself helps to remove fluid, but if the muscles of the leg are in good shape they will pump better all the time and be less likely to permit significant fluid accumulation.

One very pleasant activity—sitting in a warm bath—has been scientifically shown to help the body rid itself of edema. In a study published two years ago in the *Journal of Obstetrics and Gynecology*, the authors compared bed rest, immersion in a bathtub with water up to the waist, and immersion in a special tank up to the shoulders for their ability to reduce edema in women who were in the last three months of pregnancy. The immersion tank worked the best, but the bath produced about 50 percent more water loss than mere bed rest. Blood pressure went down, too. These techniques provide a significant de-stressing effect as well. Other studies show that a warm bath at night improves the quality of sleep.

Swimming has an even greater effect on retained fluid; this is why it is the best exercise for women with fluid retention problems. For the person fortunate enough to have a swimming pool, a period of quiet immersion after active swimming can further increase fluid removal. Baths and swimming pools help get rid of fluid because the pressure of the water on the legs tends to push the fluid back into the circulation and then to the kidney for elimination.

One of the most unpleasant symptoms associated with fluid retention is bloating, a sense of uncomfortable fullness in the abdomen. Bloating may temporarily make some clothes uncomfortably tight. Bloating is not actually due to fluid retention directly. Unfortunately, this common problem has received no real study. It is likely that it results from the effects of progesterone. Just as this hormone relaxes the smooth muscle of the uterus, it probably does the same to the smooth muscle of the intestine. The intestines expand, stretching the abdominal wall and thereby producing tight clothes and discomfort. Constipation may occur for the same reason. Once the progesterone influence is over, the intestines resume their normal caliber and the discomfort is over. But this can take a few days. While laxatives are widely condemned, their occasional use is harmless. A reasonable limit is two doses per cycle. Stronger laxatives like phenolphthalein (Ex-Lax®, Sandoz Consumer) and biscodyl (Dulcolax®, CIBA) are best avoided. Long-term excessive use of phenolphthalein can injure the colon and cause it to stop functioning. Laxatives seem to cause weight loss, but that is because they increase water loss from the intestine. Used repeatedly, they have some of the same problems as diuretics: depletion of potassium and other essential elements. The best measures to combat bloating are similar to those for water retention: proper eating and exercise. Foods high in animal fat slow the movement of the gastro-intestinal tract and make bloating worse. Avoiding beans and other foods that cause gas is a good idea, too. Finally, it may be best to simply accept the need to wear looser clothes at these times, annoying as it is to have to do so.

What was the outcome of Elizabeth's case? Her use of the very strong diuretic furosemide was making her problem worse. She did not seem very interested in lifestyle changes or a plan to taper the furosemide she was taking. It became apparent that she wanted an easy cure. This is not unreasonable; we all want to continue to live our lives in the ways we like. But in the case of idiopathic edema, there is no cure unless one is willing to change the factors that are making the natural tendency to fluid retention so much worse. The most I could do for Elizabeth was to prescribe a potassium supplement so that she would not be dangerously depleted of this mineral.

Then there was Miriam. She came from another state to see me because of leg swelling that caused her, as she put it, "truly terrible misery" most of the month. Miriam had been on diuretics for several years and gradually had increased the dose until she was on 40 mg of furosemide a day at the time I saw her. This is a whopping dose of a very powerful drug. I explained that there was no way out for her other than stopping the furosemide, although she would have even worse fluid retention for some weeks; in effect, Miriam would have to get worse before she would get better. Miriam was honest in relating her fear of what would happen, how she would look, and how she would feel without any diuretic. Since her job required her to be on her feet much of the day, any increase in the discomfort she experienced in her legs would make it difficult for her to do her work, and the standing would itself exacerbate the swelling. Together we worked out a plan. Miriam would take a medical leave from her job and start withdrawing from the diuretic in the hospital, so that help would be available if the swelling became greater than she could tolerate. (This was some years ago, before insurance companies became as hard-nosed as they are now about hospitalizations.)

Off furosemide, Miriam did progressively gain weight—all of which was fluid, not fat—and she did develop quite a degree of edema of her legs. The highest gain weight she experienced was 12 pounds. This amount of fluid retention is as great as can occur with heart or kidney disease. Miriam was very uncomfortable and struggled to keep up her morale. She dreaded being weighed in the morning and was only partly cheered up by my assurance that the weight was only water and that she would soon be rid of it. Then, after about a week, the swelling stopped getting worse, and in a few more days, it started to decrease. At this point, I sent her home with another exhortation to resist the temptation to swallow furosemide again.

Miriam stuck to it and put up with her swollen legs. While never a voracious salt eater, she now had to avoid not only the salt shaker but other foods she'd often enjoyed, such as french fries and pizza. Her efforts paid off. The extra fluid gradually went away. She could again wear slacks that had been too tight when she had come home from the hospital. She made an effort to exercise. Still there was some mild weight gain and a puffy feeling in the days before her period. She doubted she would be secure wearing shorts in the summer, despite my assurance that her legs did not look thick at all. But Miriam told me that she was relieved to be off the diuretic. "I knew that years more on a strong medicine like that was not going to be good for me. Sometimes when my weight is up a pound or two, I'm tempted to take the furosemide again. But I know I am much healthier now and that is most important."

Chapter Nine

•

Hormones, Mood, Energy, and Lifestyle

Energy and Mood

Millions of people do not feel well much or most of the time. Many of the reasons for this are obvious: excessive stress at work, family or relationship problems, financial insecurity, and a variety of chronic illness. However, there are a group of overlapping conditions that are extremely common and that seem to affect women primarily. They are related to hormones, although they are not entirely caused by them. The emphasis in this chapter will be on describing these problems, as well as on giving sound, practical recommendations on relieving them. I have said sound recommendations because this is, unfortunately, an area in which a great deal of questionable advice has been promulgated.

Melanie had a demanding job as a buyer for women's clothes at a department store. She faced many deadlines and had to put in extra hours at short notice. If sales slowed, the pressures on her increased even more. Despite this, Melanie had always done well when under pressure. She'd been married for two years. Her husband's job as a management consultant was equally demanding, and at times he would be out of town on an assignment and be home only for the weekend. Because Melanie was so busy, she said she didn't mind this. She felt she and her husband had an excellent relationship.

A few months before coming to see me, Melanie had noticed her energy level declining. "Now it is all I can do to finish my work each day. Driving home is an effort, and when I get home I just lie around and then go to bed. My husband would like to go out more, but I'm not up to it. I don't understand it. I've always liked my job, and I used to have plenty of energy. Now none of it is fun. I'm just too tired." Melanie's fatigue had not begun with the flu or any other illness; it just came on gradually.

In part due to her erratic schedule, Melanie ate irregularly. She almost never had breakfast, and when busy at work she would not eat there either. She'd followed an exercise program but stopped it about six months earlier. The decline in her energy had become very depressing to Melanie. "We'd talked about starting a family in a year or two, but I don't see how I can. I just wouldn't have the energy to give a child the attention it needs."

Melanie's problem was in part nutritional. She ate on no fixed schedule and used coffee to keep herself going when she felt herself slowing down. When she went out with her husband after an arduous week at work, she often had two or three glasses of wine to help herself relax, although she did not often drink during the week. The answer for her was in part to eat frequently in small amounts and to limit her coffee to one cup at the beginning of her day. This helped but did not completely restore her energy. She also gradually learned to control the demands of her job so that they were not as depleting. At first, she resisted the idea that her lifestyle was part of the problem. "I've always lived this way since I started working. I really do not think this is why I am so tired." Gradually I was able to convince her to try these modifications, and she found that they helped. She still feels tired at times, as people with demanding jobs often do. But she is not too tired to enjoy herself.

Annette was seventeen, and I had known her for the five years I had followed her for a thyroid condition. Now in her senior year of high school, she had become so tired that most afternoons she didn't see her friends but simply went home and took a nap. After dinner, she would do her homework and then go to bed. "I'm very worried about her," Annette's mother told me. "This is just not her. She's always had lots of friends whom she enjoyed, and now she says she's too tired to see them."

Annette also was vice president of her class and played in the band. She planned to go on to college but now was afraid she would not have the energy. Still she maintained her straight-A average. Her mother doubted she was under any stress because she had always enjoyed school and done well at it. Her nutrition was fine, and she got enough sleep, perhaps more than enough. She'd had mononucleosis a year earlier but had bounced back after three weeks of feeling weak.

One possibility was that Annette's thyroid condition might be out of control, but blood tests clearly showed that her dose of thyroid medication was correct for her. She and her mother were totally puzzled by her condition. Although it was hard for them to see it, Annette was simply doing too much and needed to make decisions about what was truly important to her and what was not.

Cassandra had come to see me because of mood swings. She was the mother of three children and worked as a secretary. "Sometimes I don't know why my husband puts up with me.

He tells me I'm great most of the month but the rest . . . He is tactful about it, but I know I can be very hard to get along with. And I take it out on my kids too. Is there anything you can do for me? Do you think I have PMS?"

Since she was moody and irritable mainly in the week before she got her period, Cassandra had already made the link to her menstrual cycle. In some women with PMS, the relationship is not as obvious. Cassandra's PMS was relatively mild. It did not threaten her relationships, but she felt very guilty about the way she sometimes behaved. As we talked, I found no reason to think that she had any particular anger toward her husband or children that was being blamed on PMS. The problem seemed to be purely hormonal. In addition to her mood changes, Cassandra also had some mild fluid retention during her period. I prescribed spironolactone for her because it has been reported to even out mood swings in women with PMS. While spironolactone does not always work—no single treatment for PMS works for all women who have it—there was considerable benefit in Cassandra's case. While she still felt irritable or low at times, these were infrequent and tolerable. Family life became calmer and more enjoyable for Cassandra.

Physician attitudes toward conditions like these vary. Not all doctors are sympathetic. It is easy to retreat before the complexity of mood and energy problems, with their inter-mixture of physical and mental factors, by denying them any reality at all. Some physicians consider them imaginary. This is obviously not so, but our scientific medical tradition, for all its great accomplishments, is not yet very effective in under-standing problems in which mind and body influence each other. It is much better at the purely physical or psychological. Mood and energy are very subtle functions, much more so that the heartbeat or even the secretions of the pituitary gland. Scientific understanding of these conditions is limited, but this does not provide an excuse to ignore them. At the same time, nothing is served by pretending that our understanding is more complete than it really is.

Terms you may have heard for the conditions discussed in this chapter include PMS, chronic fatigue, hypoglycemia, and low blood pressure. These conditions have common features: low mood, irritability or sensitivity, decreased energy, and uncomfortable physical symptoms. I have described them separately because they are usually considered different conditions. However, the distinctions in the lives of real people are not so clear. The treatments differ in some respects but are generally similar. For this reason, it seems artificial to separate them completely. You may recognize a situation like your own in one of the syndromes, or you may have some of the symptoms of more than one. This is not something to be troubled over. The important thing is to get relief, and this does not require that your condition be placed neatly in one or another category.

Low mood is a feature common to all these conditions, which tend to involve an element of depression. This does not mean depression in the sense of the word that is usually intended, which implies a strong feeling of sadness or discouragement. As a medical term, depression is a condition in which one may feel sad, but just as important are other features, such as decreased energy, appetite change, difficulty sleeping, and a sense of not being up to life's challenges. Some people have these symptoms of depression without feeling very sad.

Depression is very common and its incidence increases with age. Not everyone who is depressed feels blue, but all have decreased energy and discouragement. Depression can be due to unhappy events in one's life, but more often no particular cause can be found. Considerable evidence indicates that the cause of this so-called endogenous depression is biochemical. Certain chemicals in the brain are depleted, and a lowering of mood and energy results. This kind of depression responds to medications that readjust the balance of brain chemicals and restore normal levels of those that are depleted. The biochemical changes of depression can occur without anything bad happening in one's life. This kind of depression is hard to recognize as what it is; this is doubly unfortunate because it responds very well to treatment. Keep in mind in what follows that when I refer to depression I refer to the biochemical form.

While this chapter will cover treatment in detail, including the use of hormones and medications, it is also full of advice about diet and lifestyle. How you live and eat does have a great impact on how you feel, and I have tried to present the information in a realistic way. For example I have not recommended that everyone eat a vegetarian or extremely low-fat diet, even though there is considerable evidence that this is the healthiest way to live. The emphasis here is on those aspects of diet and lifestyle that may be contributing to your not feeling well, and on suggesting the simplest possible ways to improve them. What is presented is practical rather than ideal.

Premenstrual Syndrome (PMS)

The term "PMS" has become part of our culture and seems to need no definition. However, the popular use of the term and the medical use are not entirely the same. In popular use, PMS refers to any mood changes or other disturbing symptoms occurring at a particular point during the menstrual cycle. The medical definition is stricter: A woman is considered to have PMS only if she had the same symptoms recurrently at the same part of her cycle, usually the late luteal or premenstrual phase, but occasionally also around the time of ovulation. If she has symptoms at other times but they are worse before her period, this is not counted as PMS.

I consider this definition too restrictive. Many women who do have mild changes other times find them much more troubling before their period; they need help also. In discussing

PMS, therefore, I will consider all situations in which a woman has problems with her feelings during certain times of her cycle. The symptoms usually consist of mood shifts, which can be quite sudden, as when something of no importance will cause her to burst into tears; increased irritability; or unusual sensitivity. In the latter case, an innocent remark will cause unexpected and possibly unreasonable anger. Other mental effects of PMS include anxiety, decreased energy, aggression, and difficulty sleeping. Physical symptoms include bloating, fluid retention and weight gain, increased hunger, especially for salty or sweet foods, breast discomfort, constipation or diarrhea, and headache.

Many women have mild degrees of one or more of these symptoms but do not find that their life is interfered with. They really do not have PMS. However, when such changes interfere with work or relationships, the situation is more serious, and it is worth trying to obtain relief, either through lifestyle change or through medical treatment.

Usually PMS becomes a problem when women are in their thirties. Younger women are much more likely to have menstrual cramps, but are less likely to have mood changes. During their thirties the demands on many women greatly increase in the form of small children and demanding careers, and symptoms that could be more readily tolerated before may become less easy to handle then.

Hormonal theories of PMS have been popular but controversial. Doctor Katharina Dalton at University College Hospital, London, made the concept of PMS common knowledge; she felt that it was due to deficiency of progesterone during the second half of the cycle. More recent research has not confirmed the idea that PMS is always due to progesterone deficiency. Several studies have compared hormone levels in women with PMS to levels in other women who do not have it. These have not found any difference in luteal progesterone levels, or the amount of estrogen or prolactin. Does this mean that PMS is imaginary? Of course it does not. It merely means that we have not yet identified the chemical events involved. It is very obvious that hormones are involved in PMS. The problem is that researchers have been looking in the wrong place. The important hormonal events of PMS are not in the blood, where it is easiest to measure hormones, but in the brain, where it is impossible to measure them in humans. And PMS is clearly a uniquely human problem. But animal research does give us some clues.

Estrogen, progesterone, androgens, and thyroid hormone all have specific receptors inside the brain to which they bind. This enables them to interact with specific regions of DNA (the hereditary material) and influence brain function. Estrogen even alters the structure of certain brain cells so that they interconnect more richly to others. As Doctor Bruce McEwen of Rockefeller University puts it, "estrogen rewires the brain." Estrogen also affects the sensitivity of the brain to certain of the chemicals that conduct impulses between nerve cells, or neurotransmitters. Progesterone has been less fully studied, but it also acts on the brain in distinctive ways. It is no more surprising that hormones can cause mood changes than that they should cause breast tenderness or menstrual cramps. The exact details, however, of how mood is changed by estrogen and progesterone remain to be discovered.

What is useful to women with PMS about this research is that it shows quite clearly that hormone effects on the brain are not imaginary. It also shows why studies done by sampling hormone levels in the blood have missed the point. The differences between women with PMS and those who breeze through their premenstrual days must lie in the brain and its chemical response to estrogen and progesterone. This can account for why progesterone helps some women but not others. In some, the brain's progesterone receptors may be less sensitive and need some extra progesterone, while in others the problem may lie in a different biochemical aspect of mood regulation. I am offering speculations, but the basic point—that PMS is a problem in brain response to estrogen and progesterone—seems inescapable.

All the mental effects of PMS are ones that can occur at other times, without relation to the menstrual cycle. The changes of the cycle just bring out unpleasant feelings that might occur anyway. It seems likely, then, that the hormones or their receptors do not so much cause low mood or irritability as interfere with how the brain regulates mood. There is some evidence that in women with PMS, endorphins (natural opiates that confer a sense of well-being and comfort) are lower in the second half of the cycle. Estrogen increases endorphins in the first part of the cycle, and it is possible that in some women PMS represents a lack of endorphins needed to maintain mood because their brain requires more estrogen than it gets in order to maintain endorphin production throughout the cycle.

Not everyone feels that mood changes related to the menstrual cycle are bad. Some women feel that the variation in mood and thought during the 28 days of the menstrual cycle enrich a woman's life and that the more difficult feelings of the days before menstruation should not be suppressed. They suggest that these days, in which the body is being prepared for pregnancy, can be a time of enhanced reflection and creativity. A somewhat different view is that the feelings of anger or sadness occurring in PMS are true feelings caused by unsatisfactory aspects of the woman's condition. Some go so far as to say that the changed personality of PMS is the woman's true personality. Each idea might be true for different women.

I think these unconventional ideas contain some truth, but not the only truth. Some of the anger or sadness may be real, and hormones may simply bring them to the surface. If you have PMS, it is worth considering this possibility. If so, what you need is not hormonal or other medication, but to find a way to correct what is frustrating you, whether it be job, family, or other aspects of your life. Hormones may be the problem, or they may simply be making another problem worse. Often counseling and medical treatment can both be helpful.

Fatigue in Healthy Adults

Scientific medicine has all but ignored the issue of human energy, which is something quite different from the forms of energy studied in physics. To be sure, our bodies need those kinds of energy. Without a constant supply of new chemical energy in the form of food, none of our tissues can continue to function. But what we experience as energy in our lives is something different. To give a simple example, overeating high calorie foods gives the body an abundance of chemical energy but usually leaves us feeling tired and decidedly nonenergetic. Psychological problems can deplete energy; when that is the case, the treatment is psychological rather than purely medical.

While Western medicine has not concerned itself with energy, the opposite is the case with Oriental systems. Both Chinese and Indian Ayurvedic medicine have elaborate theories describing energy flow in the body and how blockages in them can cause disease. Acupuncture is based on stimulating and balancing various energies and is the primary treatment for low-energy problems in China. The Ayurvedic system is related to Yoga and conceives of the body in terms of seven or more energy centers called chakras, with channels connecting them. The two systems are different in detail but share a concern with energy and its localization in the body. While Western medicine is now trying to learn from these systems, which are thousands of years old, such studies are still in their infancy. This makes it hard to recommend Oriental medicine to American women who are having energy problems. Studies of non-Western medical systems may add greatly to our understanding of human energy, but this lies in the future. I would not advise against trying such approaches, but I do recommend being prudent. Be seen by a Western-style doctor first to be sure there is no identifiable disease causing your symptoms. Do not take any herbs unless you can be sure they do not have serious side effects, and, if you have acupuncture, be certain the needles are sterile and disposable.

Efforts have been made to understand chronic fatigue in scientific terms, but the studies have not yielded clear answers. In the past, low energy was attributed to a variety of causes, including subtle underactivity of the thyroid or adrenal gland, hypoglycemia, and low blood pressure.

Energy and Hormones— The Thyroid and Adrenal Glands

Profound underactivity of the thyroid can produce both sluggishness and weight gain (although only mild weight gain). Until the 1970s, hypothyroidism was a popular explanation for chronic fatigue, especially when it was combined with a tendency to be overweight. Many women were placed on thyroid hormone preparations because of these symptoms. What has made hypothyroidism less popular as an explanation for these problems is the invention of extremely accurate tests for measuring the function of the thyroid gland. It turned out that most of those suspected of having mild hypothyroidism did not have it. Currently the supersensitive TSH assay is most helpful because it can detect beginning underactivity of the thyroid at a stage before any symptoms have occurred. (TSH is the pituitary hormone that stimulates the thyroid. If the thyroid is slowing down, TSH goes up because the pituitary gland recognizes that the thyroid needs more stimulation.) It is important to have your thyroid tested if you have an energy problem, but it is likely to be normal.

If you do turn out to have an underactive thyroid, treatment is simply taking the thyroid hormone thyroxine (also called levothyroxine) in pill form. Dose is important; too little will leave you still mildly hypothyroid, while too much will cause hyperthyroidism. As we have gotten better at measuring thyroid function, standard doses have been revised downward. For most women, the correct dose is 0.112 mg daily. This is too much for some women; I have adult patients whose proper dose is as low as 0.088 mg. A few need more, 0.125 or occasionally 0.150 mg, but it is rare to need this much. Long-term excess of thyroid hormone causes loss of calcium from the bones. If you are on thyroid, be sure your TSH, as measured by the supersensitive assay, is in the normal range. If not, have your dose adjusted. You will not function at your best if you do not have a normal level of thyroid hormone. There are two reliable preparations of levothyroxine: Synthroid® (Boots Pharmaceuticals) and Levothroid® (Forest Pharmaceuticals). Generics are unreliable and should be avoided. Once your dose has been regulated, it is best to stay with the same brand; different preparations may not be absorbed to exactly the same degree.

Surprisingly, low energy is more likely to be due to overactivity of the thyroid than to underactivity. Excessive levels of thyroid hormone stimulate chemical energy production to the point where the body cannot use it efficiently and fatigue results. Grave's disease is the most common cause of hyperthyroidism and is at least four times as common in women as in men. It is not unusual for it to be detected accidentally when tests looking for hypothyroidism are done because of chronic fatigue. Other symptoms of overactivity of the thyroid are nervousness, being hot all the time, excessive sweating, and bulging of the eyes. It may cause lower grades in children and reduced work efficiency in adults. Grave's disease can be treated with medication, radioactive iodine, or surgery. Radioiodine, which has been studied carefully for several decades, is both the most effective treatment and the safest. Surgery is sometimes carried out but can have significant complications, including paralysis of the vocal cords.

Adrenal insufficiency, called Addison's disease, is quite rare. It causes fatigue, low levels of sodium and high potassium, and deepening of skin pigmentation. These changes are due to the body's lack of cortisol and aldosterone. The late President John F. Kennedy had Addison's disease, which accounted for his tanned look. While subtle adrenal underactivity might seem plausible as an explanation for fatigue, there is no evidence that this condition actually exists. Some women with chronic fatigue are told they have a slight decrease in the function of their adrenals and are placed on cortisone.

Cortisone does increase energy in the short term because, like adrenaline, it is involved in preparing the body for the increased energy expenditure required in a situation of danger. However, the increase in energy is short term. If cortisone is continued, energy is produced by the breakdown of healthy tissue, especially muscle, bone, and skin. Taking cortisone or equivalent hormones if you do not need them is dangerous. They have no place in the treatment of chronic fatigue because of their eventual serious side effects. If you have been told you have mild adrenal deficiency, I suggest that you get another opinion from an experienced endocrinologist.

While hormonal problems such as thyroid or adrenal dysfunction can cause fatigue, fewer than 1 percent of women with chronic fatigue have these conditions.

Infection, Immunity, and Fatigue

Recently research has looked for problems with the immune system in women with chronic fatigue. It is important to realize that the researchers have defined chronic fatigue syndrome (CFS) in a very specific way. Many women who have chronic low energy do not meet the criteria for CFS, and so the findings may not apply to them. As strictly defined, CFS begins with an acute viral illness resembling a cold or flu. After the acute symptoms go away in a week or so, there is a persistence of the fatigue or weak feeling typical of viral illnesses like the "flu." In CFS this fatigue persists for weeks or months. Sudden onset with a viral infection is the most important defining characteristic of CFS. If you are chronically tired but the condition began gradually and did not start with a definite viral illness, then you do not have the specific CFS condition that I am discussing in this section, and your fatigue is not likely to be due to infection or immune dysfunction.

Several infectious organisms have been studied for a role in producing CFS. The first was yeast, or *candida albicans* (also called monilia). Several books popularized the idea that yeast, which normally colonizes the vagina, can spread to other parts of the body and produce a hidden infection. Treatment consisted in avoiding foods that contain fungus, such as cheese, and taking antibiotics, such as nystatin (various manufacturers), that are effective against candida. This is a different situation from the common vaginal yeast infections, in which the problem is only in the vagina and is easily eliminated by proper treatment. Carefully done studies have not confirmed the idea that yeast infection can spread into the body and cause chronic fatigue in otherwise healthy people.

The infectious agent that has been most studied with respect to CFS is the Epstein-Barr virus (EBV), which causes infectious mononucleosis. There is no doubt that some people take a long time to recover from mono. Many people with CFS do have evidence of EBV infection, but some do not. Another virus some think is involved with CFS is herpes virus type 6. Enteroviruses, which are normal in the gastro-intestinal tract but not elsewhere, have been found in the muscle tissue of some people with CFS. One study has linked CFS in some farm children to drinking unpasteurized milk. It seems likely that chronic viral infection or mild deficiencies of the immune system can cause CFS, but a clear picture has yet to emerge. It is very difficult to prove a viral cause in an individual person with CFS. The viruses linked to it are very common ones, and it is hard to tell when they have caused the fatigue or are there because of an unrelated infection.

A variety of abnormalities of immune function have been found in people with CFS. One study found low immunoglobulins and a beneficial effect of intravenous gamma globulin. Others have found defects in the function of NK cells, which kill infecting organisms, and a lessening of the normal increase of lymphocytes with stimulation.

If you suddenly developed tiredness right after a flu-like illness, it is worth going to a physician who specializes in infectious diseases and being evaluated. The diagnosis is complex, and the knowledge of a specialist is needed. If your energy problem developed gradually and did not begin suddenly after an illness or infection, immune deficiency is probably not involved, and treatment directed at infection or the immune system is not likely to be helpful to you. Please note that chronic fatigue that is not due to infection or immune problems is just as real but simply has a different cause.

For women with chronic fatigue, there seem to be two factors involved. The first is a physical factor, such as a viral illness, hypoglycemia, low blood pressure, or PMS, but equally important is a condition of being under a high level of demand. Fatigue has always been common in college students because studies and social activities are far more taxing than they were in high school. (Lately, however, the demands on high school students have increased, and chronic fatigue seems to be becoming more common in teenagers.) American cultural ideas about illness may make it worse because we emphasize being independent and recovering from illness as quickly as possible. We see an example of this in current trends in hospitalization. After hysterectomy, a major operation by anyone's accounting, women were once allowed two weeks of hospital recovery and are now lucky to get three days. The reason given for this is cost containment, but it seems to me also that American culture has gotten less tolerant of any situation in which physical problems limit energy or activity. This is especially hard on women, whose work day rarely ends when they get home in the evening. My point is that the body sometimes needs respite from the demands of modern life, and that respite may be almost impossible to get. One result can be chronic fatigue.

Treatment of chronic fatigue is directed against the two factors I have mentioned. If a physical abnormality can be identified, it should be treated. Most often, a specific cause cannot be identified or, in the case of viral infections, there is no specific treatment. The need for an extended recovery period should be accepted, and unnecessary activities should be dropped. However, withdrawing from all activities is inadvisable. Rest should be adequate but not excessive, because this only leads to more tiredness. Returning to full activity is like resuming a sport after a long period out of training. It should be done gradually but progressively. Attention to lifestyle is very important (see below). Depression is a factor in many chronic fatigue states. This does not mean that chronic fatigue is caused by depression, but depression is a component of it that responds very well to treatment. Of medical treatments, fluoxitine (Prozac®) is most likely to be effective. It seems to correct the chemical changes in the brain that causes the abnormal energy and mood.

Hypoglycemia

Some basic facts about metabolism will make hypoglycemia easy to understand. Our body chemistry is very different in the fasted and fed states. Eating induces the release of insulin, which helps move the breakdown of food (glucose and amino acids) into the cells. Insulin also stops the release of glucose and fat by the liver. These responses help the body store food energy that is not needed immediately. Once food is fully digested, however, no more nutrients enter the blood from the intestine; the liver and muscles must now release glucose and other nutrients so that levels are maintained in the blood and the tissues are not starved. The brain is most sensitive to lack of glucose, because it cannot make its own and is thus dependant on a steady supply from the bloodstream. So great is the need of the brain for glucose that unconsciousness occurs within a few minutes if glucose levels dip very low.

In the fasting state, insulin levels must drop so that the liver can break down its starch stores to release glucose. The body's emergency protection against low blood glucose is adrenaline, and this hormone is usually released when blood sugar drops too low. Adrenaline not only lifts levels of glucose in the blood, it also makes the heart pound and gives rise to a strong sense of anxiety and danger. This is part of the normal response that prepares the body for fight or flight by mobilizing glucose for energy. However, in our normal lives, the fight or flight aspects of the action of adrenaline are irrelevant and merely serve to cause a feeling of impending doom that can be very frightening.

In most people, these metabolic processes function smoothly, and one is never aware of them. However, some people have difficulty switching from the fed to the fasted state. In extreme cases, blood glucose drops very low and unconsciousness or even convulsions result. This is true hypoglycemia and occurs when blood glucose levels drop below 40 to 45 mg/dl. The brain simply cannot get enough fuel when glucose levels in the blood are this low. (There is some individual variation in how low the blood glucose level must go to cause difficulty.) Hypoglycemia severe enough to cause convulsions or unconsciousness is quite rare; it may result from a tumor making too much insulin or a problem in the pituitary or adrenal gland that prevents it from making enough growth hormone or cortisol. These are potentially life-threatening disorders that require careful diagnosis and treatment by a physician experienced with them, usually an endocrinologist.

When otherwise healthy people are told they have hypoglycemia, it is usually not this severe problem but a relative hypoglycemia, in which blood glucose levels stay in the normal range but some discomfort is felt when they are in the lower part of the normal range. Blood glucose levels go down to the 50s or occasionally the upper 40s, but only for very brief periods. Symptoms are those of hunger, but more so: anxiety, lightheadedness, dizziness, lack of mental clarity. Often adrenaline is released, which produces a feeling of fear as well as sweating and palpitations. This form of hypoglycemia is really a mild abnormality in making the transition to the fasting state.

This relative hypoglycemia usually occurs in women who are slender and often do not have strong hunger feelings, so that they often miss meals or eat very little. Some feel hungry but do not eat because of concern about weight control. In women with hypoglycemia, the change in metabolism to the fasting state occurs only after glucose levels have fallen enough to give rise to some degree of discomfort. When tested, their blood glucose is usually at the low normal limit of about 50 mg/dl or sometimes slightly lower. Sometimes these levels are mistakenly interpreted as abnormal because doctors usually have become used to levels in people suspected of having diabetes, who have much higher levels that are therefore less healthy. The problem in relative hypoglycemia is not the blood sugar levels but the body's uncomfortable reaction to them.

Low Blood Pressure

Decades ago, low blood pressure was thought to be an abnormality, and the statement "You have low blood pressure" caused people to worry, although what was bad about low blood pressure was never very clear. By the time I was in medical school, the teaching was that there is no such thing as low blood pressure because many studies have shown that the lower someone's blood pressure, the greater their life expectancy. In this sense, low blood pressure is a sign of health.

More recently, some studies, including a very large one on over 10,000 government office workers in London, have shown that men and women with low systolic blood pressure were more likely to have dizziness and feel tired. The finding is surprising; low blood pressure is a sign of health. We normally expect what is healthy to make us feel better and more energetic.

Many healthy young women have blood pressures between 85 to 95 systolic over 50 to 60 diastolic. This level can be considered low, but most women with pressures in this range feel fine. However, some do not. Most women with low blood pressure are slender and have low intakes of food, salt, and water. They often skip meals when they are busy or nervous. These traits resemble those of women who have relative hypoglycemia. There is no treatment for low blood pressure because raising the blood pressure would have an unfavorable effect on long-term health. (Some people with extremely low pressures may nearly faint when they sit or stand up; this rare orthostatic hypotension can be treated.)

What should you do if you have low blood pressure? First of all, be glad; you are most likely in a very low-risk group for cardiovascular disease. Medication is not necessary or appropriate. I recommend you follow the advice I give later in this chapter about lifestyle, especially eating frequently and drinking enough water. You probably should not limit your salt intake too much because this will tend to lower your blood volume and therefore your blood pressure.

Hormones and Medical Treatments for PMS

There is no question that PMS is due to hormones. However, despite claims made by some doctors, my experience and that of many other endocrinologists and of gynecologists has been that hormonal treatments do not often work very well. The problem is that, while hormones are clearly involved in PMS, it is often impossible to pin down just what in a woman's hormonal pattern is causing her symptoms. One or two hormone measurements done at the time of a visit may not be at all representative of what is happening at other times. Furthermore, as I have explained, the hormones that cause PMS are those in the brain, not those in the blood.

Without treatment, PMS has an intractable quality. No matter what is happening, or what the demands of work or relationship are, depression or irritability occurs and interferes, often with what is most important in a woman's life. Willpower is seemingly of no help, although women with PMS do sometimes rearrange things so as to avoid scheduling important occasions during the part of the cycle when mood changes are a problem. Even here, however, since PMS varies from cycle to cycle, it is not always possible to avoid important matters during the difficult part. Indeed this variability of PMS is one of its most frustrating features.

Modern life makes it almost impossible to live by our natural biological rhythms. One hundred years ago, middle- and upper-class women were not expected to be active during their periods; to take to their beds when not feeling well was perfectly acceptable. This is no longer acceptable; indeed the idea of resting when not feeling well has been left behind in the busy pace of modern life. Work and family responsibilities make bed rest for PMS impossible. Nor would most women want to withdraw for a part of each month. But the point is still valid; the demands of contemporary life make the normal shifting of moods and energy level harder to deal with.

Women with PMS usually have a biological vulnerability to low mood or irritability. This tendency is brought out by the hormonal changes of the menstrual cycle. Hormones trigger low mood rather than cause it. The regulation of mood is subtle and complex. Many people have a tendency to feel blue from time to time, but others do not. Some even maintain their cheerfulness in the face of terrible events. There are cultural factors at work here, too. Because Americans believe we can and should change our circumstances for the better, we are more likely to be frustrated when we cannot. The Chinese, who regard misfortune as inevitably a large part of life, often are less depressed by it because their expectations are lower. I am not saying that they do not mind, only that depression is less a part of their way of reacting.

There are two possible medical approaches to treatment of PMS. One is to alter the hormones during the cycle or to alter their action. The second is to counteract the tendency to low mood. There is also a non-medical approach, which is to alter lifestyle and environmental factors that adversely affect mood.

I wish I could say that there is a scientific method for picking out which of these treatments is most likely to be effective. There isn't. There are often clues as to which will help, but some period of trial and error is almost inevitable. Each person's pattern is a little different, and what helps greatly for one woman may do almost nothing for someone else. This is one reason why there are so many strong viewpoints in the field. Each physician or other practitioner who treats women with PMS tends to develop a patient population whose PMS responds to his or her favorite treatment. This tends to reinforce a sense of certainty that *the* answer to PMS has been found. Anyone who reads the medical or lay literature on this subject is well aware of the strong claims that are typically made. Yet most women who have PMS know only too well that for them the solution is not so simple.

I think that realizing that it will take some time to find the best treatment is the first step toward getting help. Otherwise the depression of having PMS in the first place is only made worse by disappointment when a much-vaunted treatment fails to solve the problem. It is also something that, as a doctor, I want my patients with PMS to know. If the first treatments tried do not work, it is not necessarily lack of knowledge or concern on the part of the physician, but the confusing and variable nature of PMS itself. If you seek medical help for PMS, it is important to have a physician who not only takes the problem seriously but is willing to take the time to work out an individualized treatment with you. Some physicians who work in this area are committed to certain treatments. If these work, it is fine, but if they do not, the physician may not be the best one for you. At the same time, it is reasonable to give a treatment an adequate trial before giving up.

Progesterone is the treatment first advocated for PMS. This has always been something of a problem since natural proges-terone itself is not made by any of the major pharmaceutical companies. It is available from a special pharmacy by mail order; (see page 479).

Since micronized progesterone is now available and is satis-factorily absorbed, there is no reason to use the older supposi-tories. The oral dose is one to three 100-mg capsules each day during the luteal phase, which is the last two weeks of the cycle. The best dose for most women is 100 mg twice a day; doses of 300 mg daily or higher can cause tiredness. You can determine when your luteal phase is by doing basal body temperatures or just by the calendar, especially if your periods are regular within a few days each month. If you are doing it by calendar, simply start 14 days before you expect the first day of your period or a day or two before symptoms usually start. Using progesterone in this way does not provide contraception. Progesterone does seem to help some women considerably, but I recommend it only if other approaches have not worked for you simply because the other approaches have a higher probability of working.

Spironolactone which I discussed in Chapters Six and Eight is helpful for some women with PMS, especially those with fluid-retention problems. Some of the women for whom I had prescribed it because of an androgenic disorder have told me it helped their premenstrual moodiness, even though I had not mentioned this as a possible effect. Although birth control pills can make menstrual-cycle mood problems worse, a few women feel better when they take them. The prolactin-lowering drug bromocryptine (Parlodel®) has been used in PMS on the theory that prolactin causes some of the symptoms. This drug causes dizziness and nausea in some women and is best avoided unless you need it for a prolactin problem. Nor do I recommend clonidine (Catapres®, Boehringer Ingelheim), which causes extreme drowsiness.

For most women with PMS, however, hormonal treatments are not the most helpful ones. Except for spironolactone, they are more of a last resort. I find women usually have better relief by following the diet and lifestyle advice I have given below and, if this alone is not sufficient, using the new antidepressant fluoxitine (Prozac®). Usually the lowest dose of 20 mg once a day is enough. This is actually a more scientific treatment than progesterone because it corrects the tendency to low mood that is exacerbated late in the cycle in women with PMS. Side effects are almost nonexistent at the low dose I have recommended. It does decrease appetite, but few complain if it causes them to lose weight. Occasionally it will cause some stimulation or restlessness. It is best to take it in the morning to minimize the chance that it will interfere with sleep. Sertraline (Zoloft®, Roerig) is also effective for many women with PMS and may help insomnia. Paroxetine (Paxil®,

SmithKline Beecham) is another new antidepressant, which seems to be helpful when mood changes are accompanied by anxiety. Fluoxitine had some adverse publicity two years ago, but a careful FDA investigation did not find any substance to the concerns, which were raised in the media, of an increased suicide rate. Rather it has attracted a lot of attention because it is one of the most widely prescribed medications in the United States. Occasionally women or men taking one of these new anti-depressants experience a decrease in sexual feelings.

Although there are many older anti-depressants, most have no reason to be used in PMS. Amitriptyline (Elavil®, Stuart Pharmaceuticals) tends to cause drowsiness and increase appetite. But if you have difficulty sleeping during your PMS time but no tendency to be overweight, this may be best for you. Generally 25 to 50 mg before bed is enough. All these medications take two to three weeks to start to work; it takes this long for the chemical changes of low mood in the brain to be corrected. For this reason, they need to be taken every day, not just during the part of your cycle in which you have PMS.

Vitamin B_6 (pyridoxine) was used for many years, but there is convincing evidence that in doses of 200 mg a day or more it can cause nerve damage, which can show up as pins and needles, numbness, a crawling sensation, or oversensitivity of the skin. For this reason, it is no longer recommended. Evening primrose oil is another nutritional supplement that has been used in PMS. It contains vitamin K and essential fatty acids, including gamma-linolenic acid, which may be deficient in some women with PMS. The daily dose is two to four capsules of 500 mg each.

Which treatment is best? This is so individual that I cannot make any blanket recommendation. The first step is to correct diet and lifestyle factors that may be making matters worse. Evening primrose oil can be used to supplement the nutritional aspect. The medical treatment most likely to work is fluoxitine. Spironolactone would be the second choice, unless you also have an androgenic disorder, in which case it is probably the first one to try. If cramps or other discomfort in your female organs is part of your problem, a non-steroidal anti-inflammatory such as sulindac (Clinoril®,) or oxaprozin (Daypro®) may be a helpful addition. You should start it a day or two in your cycle before the discomfort begins and stop once the time of discomfort is over.

Diet and Lifestyle— How They Affect Mood and Energy

Being sure you are maintaining proper nutrition and lifestyle should always be the first step if mood or energy are a problem for you. Hormones and medications should be used only if these simpler, natural methods do not completely alleviate the problem. The first step is to try to avoid the unhealthy habits that overly busy and stressful lifestyles tend to promote. None of us has perfect health habits, and the purpose of this section is not to make you feel guilty but to summarize information that many have found helpful. If you feel there are changes you should make, you needn't feel they have to be done instantly. It is usually better to make changes gradually, lest the attempt to acquire better lifestyle habits becomes yet another stress.

SLEEP

The first and almost too obvious step if your energy is low is to get enough sleep. There is a tendency to think of sleeping as self-indulgence, but it is a biological necessity. The first thing to happen with mild sleep deprivation is a lowering of mood. The effects seem to be cumulative as well. Some women have trouble sleeping before their period, and the effects of this on mood are even worse if they have not gotten enough sleep earlier in the cycle. Most people need close to eight hours a night. Many can get by on less, but often at the cost of not feeling well or not functioning at best efficiency. Sleeping pills are not the answer, as they do not produce normal sleep and are potentially addicting. Aside from allowing enough time, the most important thing is to build into your schedule a period of calm before sleep. It might be reading (for pleasure, not work), a hot bath, or some other pleasant and relatively mindless activity. I am not suggesting that getting enough sleep is the complete answer to PMS, but that sleep deprivation makes any mood problem much worse. However, sleeping excessively can deplete energy; if you are getting enough sleep, more will not help. Sleep should restore you for the activities that are important to you, not replace them. Some women with chronic fatigue sleep too much and the body gradually gets out of condition, so that a normal day's activities are exhausting. The same happens after an illness that requires bed rest—it takes at least several days and sometimes longer to get back into physical condition for even ordinary activity.

WATER

Just as the demands of modern life interfere with the natural sleep-wake cycle, they also make a natural pattern of eating and drinking more difficult. Our bodies are about two-thirds water, so it is not surprising that the intake and distribution of fluid in the body is of great importance for well-being. Some women do not drink enough water and so often are slightly dehydrated. Because there is less water than the body needs, the volume of the blood is reduced, and blood does not circulate to tissues quite as effectively. The brain, being above the heart, is most affected. This can show itself as dizziness when standing up suddenly. Sometimes, however, the only symptom is vague fatigue, with no clue as to its cause.

The solution is to make sure you drink enough water. Six to eight glasses a day is usually the right amount. Any other fluid is basically water and is just as good, provided it does not have caffeine or too many calories. This is why you should not get most of your fluid from milk or juice. An adequate fluid intake will dilute your urine so it is light; a strong yellow color means you are not drinking enough.

Salt depletion can also interfere with the circulation because salt is needed to hold water. This is uncommon, except in people who use diuretics to get rid of fluid retention. Too much salt and water in the tissues can also cause fatigue or mild depression due to a feeling of discomfort or lack of energy. Waterlogged tissue is not quite normal, and a vague, hard-to-define but very real discomfort results.

NUTRITION

While the problems with mood and energy that healthy women have are not caused by dietary deficiencies, eating practices do have a major impact on well-being. The most frequent problem is not what is eaten but the timing of eating. (I am assuming you are already familiar with current dietary guidelines, get 50 percent or more of your calories from carbohydrates, and minimize your intake of saturated fat and cholesterol.) We have grown up thinking of three meals a day as a "normal" way to eat. Many women, especially those who are busy or weight-conscious, eat fewer than three meals. Some feel virtuous by regularly omitting meals. Often the timing of meals is erratic. Some people can tolerate this and feel fine, though many cannot.

If you are one of the many women who have some discomfort when your body has to make the transition from the fed to the fasted state, skipping meals will make you feel worse than is normal for you. The relative hypoglycemia is due to a lag in the body being able to make use of stored nutrients in place of food. Women who have difficulty with this metabolic adjustment are usually thin and active. They simply do not have much food stored in their bodies. Overweight women may have excessive appetites and feel very hungry if they miss meals, but they do not have a lack of stored food energy.

If you have an energy problem or relative hypoglycemia, a change in eating pattern will be very important for you. First, recognize that the idea of eating only three meals a day is cultural, not biological. It was probably devised by men, who have much more energy stored in their muscle protein and livers and rarely have the same trouble making the transition to the fasting state that slender women do. Even so, most people are better off eating six times a day, rather than only three. This suggestion scares some women because they imagine it means eating more. However, the idea is not to eat more but to eat the same amount divided into six small meals instead of three large ones. (This approach was originally developed for people with insulin-dependent diabetes because the insulin they take makes a normal change to the fasted state impossible.) A small snack is needed mid-morning, mid-afternoon, and before bed. When meals cannot be eaten on schedule— if you have a late business dinner or a date, for example—an extra small snack at the normal dinner time will help prevent symptoms. Snacks may be a piece of fruit, or a few crackers with cheese or peanut butter. Vegetables like carrots, celery, or lettuce by themselves are not enough. Eating snacks like this is not self-indulgence. It may be quite the opposite, because for many slender, busy women, it takes a special effort to eat during the day.

This kind of eating pattern is much healthier than the more usual ones. When food intake is spread out like this, there is better utilization of calories and therefore less tendency for weight gain. You feel better because your body has a more constant supply of energy from food. The need to shift several times a day to fasting state metabolism is prevented. If you have relative hypoglycemia, eating according to this pattern is the only effective treatment. If you have a tendency to fatigue, this way of eating will enable your body to use its energy more efficiently.

When relative hypoglycemia was first described, it was assumed that blood glucose dropped because of excessive insulin release following the eating of sweets. The idea that sugar makes you high and then tired or blue became widespread. This is actually a misunderstanding. Relative hypoglycemia is due not to too much insulin but to slowness of the body in shifting to fasting-state metabolism. Sugar does not precipitate hypoglycemia or a low feeling. However, if sweets are substituted for a meal, they are digested very quickly and the energy they contain is soon used up. The result is the need to shift to fasting metabolism and the tired feeling that results until glucose is released from the liver. The culprit is not sweets per se, but substituting them for a real meal or snack. People who eat candy bars instead of fruit or crackers experience this tired feeling an hour or two later.

Other than as a source of sometimes excessive calories, sweets are not harmful. If you have hypoglycemia, chronic fatigue, or PMS, the emphasis should be on eating frequent healthy foods and on not skipping meals. Simply avoiding sweets is not the solution.

EXERCISE

There is no question that regular aerobic exercise improves fitness and results in a higher energy level and tolerance for stress. At the same time, it does not solve all health problems.

Exercising too much or increasing one's running distance too rapidly can itself cause fatigue. A moderate exercise program is very helpful in maintaining energy. If you have a tendency to hypoglycemia, make sure to have a small snack, such as a piece of fruit or a glass of juice, before exercising and during exercise, if it lasts more than 30 to 45 minutes. The idea that it is bad to eat before a workout is an old superstition. The exercises that are best for health are jogging (some feel brisk walking is just as good), cycling, or swimming. Sports that require intermittent expenditure of energy, such as tennis or racquetball, are less beneficial. Weight training tones up the body but does little for cardiovascular fitness.

Yoga and Chinese exercise systems such as Tai Chi and Chi Gong were devised based on ideas for optimizing energy flows in the body and thereby promoting longevity and serenity. Many people find them helpful, and they are worth trying if you are having a problem with your energy. They are not strenuous in the way aerobic exercise is, but are challenging in a different way. Most communities have introductory courses available. As with other new activities, their benefit is not felt until you have practiced them for a while.

CAFFEINE AND ALCOHOL

I have never known anyone to feel worse as a result of eliminating alcohol or caffeine, provided they can get through the period of withdrawal. The main symptoms of caffeine withdrawal are headaches and a dull, de-energized feeling, especially in the morning. If you have a tendency to migraine, caffeine withdrawal may precipitate an attack. The solution is very simple: Eliminate caffeinated coffee slowly, no faster than one cup every one to two weeks. Your energy may decrease at first, but it will increase over its previous level once your body gets over the dependence on caffeine. The ritual of coffee drinking can continue with decaffeinated coffee. If you drink alcohol infrequently, it will not be hard for you to decrease or eliminate it, but if you have a problem with alcohol you will need to seek professional help.

Why eliminate caffeine or alcohol? Small amounts of these substances are certainly less harmful than other common habits, such as smoking or eating high-fat foods. Many studies suggest that coffee increases the risk of heart attack, but a few studies have failed to show this. With alcohol, there is no question about the serious health consequences of high intake. However, many studies suggest that a moderate amount— one or two drinks a day—may increase life expectancy. Some dispute this, suspecting that many of those studied did not drink because of health problems in which case low alcohol intake was the result rather than the cause of illness. Alcohol does raise HDL cholesterol but only the HDL-3 fraction, whereas it is the HDL-2 fraction which is beneficial. Alcohol can be a cause of high blood pressure (see page 381). Alcohol makes people feel good right after it is ingested, but they generally feel worse as the effects wear off. More than one drink usually leaves one feeling tired and uncomfortable as it wears off. Caffeine gives a feeling of warmth and energy, although efforts to increase this by drinking more coffee result in nervousness and palpitations. When caffeine wears off, after one to three hours, there is a dull feeling, a lack of energy, and, for some people, headache. This may be attributed to boredom, stress at work, or even to a health problem; in fact, it is a chemical change induced by the caffeine and its withdrawal.

The busyness of modern life does not make it easy to maintain an even mood. Adding another, artificial, and unnecessary source of mood change simply increases the complexity of adjustments that our minds and bodies must make in the course of a day. Using caffeine or alcohol means that much of the day or night will be spent in a mild withdrawal state, in which the body is not functioning in its natural way. If you have a tendency to low energy or mood swings, or if you are under unusually heavy demands, the added shifts will make it worse. Caffeine and alcohol also have diuretic effects and may deplete the body of water and minerals.

Probably most women have had one or another of the problems discussed in this chapter to a mild degree at some time in their adult lives. While there is no one perfect treatment, there are many that help. If you are lucky, the first thing you try will help. Otherwise, considerable patience and persistence may be necessary. The chances are excellent that you can get better if you give the treatments a chance.